RESEARCH REPORT

The Evolving Role of Emergency Departments in the United States

Kristy Gonzalez Morganti • Sebastian Bauhoff • Janice C. Blanchard

Mahshid Abir • Neema Iyer • Alexandria C. Smith • Joseph V. Vesely

Edward N. Okeke • Arthur L. Kellermann

Sponsored by the Emergency Medicine Action Fund

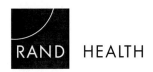

HEALTH

The research described in this report was sponsored by the Emergency Medicine Action Fund, a consortium sponsored by the American College of Emergency Physicians. The work was conducted in RAND Health, a division of the RAND Corporation.

The RAND Corporation is a nonprofit institution that helps improve policy and decisionmaking through research and analysis. RAND's publications do not necessarily reflect the opinions of its research clients and sponsors.

RAND® is a registered trademark.

© Copyright 2013 RAND Corporation

Permission is given to duplicate this document for personal use only, as long as it is unaltered and complete. Copies may not be duplicated for commercial purposes. Unauthorized posting of RAND documents to a non-RAND website is prohibited. RAND documents are protected under copyright law. For information on reprint and linking permissions, please visit the RAND permissions page (http://www.rand.org/publications/permissions.html).

Published 2013 by the RAND Corporation
1776 Main Street, P.O. Box 2138, Santa Monica, CA 90407-2138
1200 South Hayes Street, Arlington, VA 22202-5050
4570 Fifth Avenue, Suite 600, Pittsburgh, PA 15213-2665
RAND URL: http://www.rand.org/
To order RAND documents or to obtain additional information, contact
Distribution Services: Telephone: (310) 451-7002;
Fax: (310) 451-6915; Email: order@rand.org

Preface

This project was performed to develop a more complete picture of how emergency departments (EDs) contribute to the U.S. health care system. Using a mix of quantitative and qualitative methods, it explores the evolving role that hospital EDs and the personnel who staff them play in evaluating and managing complex and high-acuity patients, serving as the major portal of entry to inpatient care, and serving as "the safety net of the safety net" for patients who are unable to get care elsewhere.

This work was sponsored by the Emergency Medicine Action Fund, a consortium of emergency medicine physician organizations sponsored by the American College of Emergency Physicians. The research was conducted by RAND Health, a division of the RAND Corporation. A profile of RAND Health, abstracts of publications, and ordering information can be found at www.rand.org/health.

Table of Contents

Preface...iii

Figures..vi

Tables..vii

Executive Summary..viii

Acknowledgements...x

Abbreviations...xi

1. Introduction...1

    Trends Affecting the Evolution of Hospital EDs..1

        Overall Growth in Health Care Spending. 1

        Growing Use of Hospital EDs..2

        The Rising Cost of ED Care..2

        Efforts to Discourage Non-Urgent Use of EDs...3

        EDs as Entry Points to Inpatient Care...4

    Aims of the RAND Study...5

    Organization of This Report..6

2. Conceptual Model of ED Use..7

3. Methods..13

    Quantitative Data Sources..13

    Analytical Approach...17

    Qualitative Data Sources..21

        Emergency Physician Focus Groups..21

        Hospital Physician Focus Group...22

        Individual Interviews with Primary Care Providers...22

    Review of Qualitative Data 23

4. Findings 24

        What are the most important sources of inpatient admissions and how have they changed?............24

        What are the sources driving growth of non-elective inpatient admissions? 27

        Why are primary care physicians admitting fewer patients to hospitals? 29

        Why are patients using EDs for non-urgent care?...31

        Does a patient's insurance coverage influence likelihood of admission and his/her portal
of entry to inpatient care? 33

        Does a patient's source of primary health insurance influence his/her probability of
hospitalization from the ED? 39

        Does a patient's type of insurance influence a primary care physician's decision to send
the patient to the ED?...40

        Do plans that offer care coordination have lower rates of inpatient admission from EDs
than fee-for-service plans?..41

Are EDs playing a role in reducing preventable hospital admissions? 42

5. Discussion 49

    Assessing the Value of Emergency Department Care 49

    The Evolving Relationship Between EDs and Primary Care Providers 50

    Emergency Departments as Diagnostic Centers 51

    Do Emergency Departments Prevent Costly Inpatient Admissions? 51

    Study Limitations 53

6. Conclusions 55

    Implications for Policy 56

References 57

Figures

Figure 2.1. Conceptual Model for ED Use 7

Figure 2.2. Health Care Options for Patients 8

Figure 2.3. Causal Pathway Factors and Associated Factors for Exploring Options of Care 9

Figure 2.4. Conceptual Model for Emergency Department Care 11

Figure 4.1. Inpatient Admissions, by Source, 2003–2009 25

Figure 4.2. Share of Inpatient Admissions, by Source, 2009 26

Figure 4.3. Trends in Elective and Non-Elective Hospital Admissions, 2003–2009 27

Figure 4.4. Trends in Non-Elective Hospital Admissions, by Source, 2003–2009 28

Figure 4.5. Share of Non-Elective Inpatient Admissions, 2003–2009 29

Figure 4.6. Reasons Why Physicians Were Unable to Obtain Non-Emergency Hospital
Admissions 30

Figure 4.7. Number of Emergency Department Visits, by Year 31

Figure 4.8. Efforts to Identify Non-Emergency Department Options for Acute Care, 2003 32

Figure 4.9. Usual Source of Care and Difficulty to Contact Provider After-Hours 33

Figure 4.10. All Inpatient Admissions, by Primary Payer and Source, 2009 34

Figure 4.11. Share of All Inpatients Admitted Through the Emergency Department,
by Primary Payer, 1993–2009 35

Figure 4.12. Primary Payer for All Hospital Admissions, 1993–2009 36

Figure 4.13. Primary Payer for Inpatient Admissions Originating in Emergency
Departments, 1993–2009 37

Figure 4.14. Population Rates of Inpatient Admissions from Emergency Departments,
1999–2009 38

Figure 4.15. Population Rates of Inpatient Admission from Non–Emergency Department
Sources, 1999–2009 39

Tables

Table 3.1. National Hospital Discharge Survey Sample Sizes, 2001–2010 14

Table 3.2. Summary of Quantitative Data Sources, by Project Aim 20

Table 4.1. Emergency Department Admissions, by Payer, 2009 40

Table 4.2. AHRQ Prevention Quality Indicators Conditions and Composites............................ 43

Table 4.3. Trends in PQI-related Inpatient Admissions, by Source, 2000, 2005, and 2009........ 44

Table 4.4. PQIs Paired with Corresponding CCS Conditions 45

Table 4.5. CCS Percent Change from 2006 to 2009.. 47

Executive Summary

Emergency departments (EDs) emerged with the rise of hospital-based medicine in the aftermath of World War II. Today, they play a pivotal role in the delivery of acute ambulatory and inpatient care. As our health care system evolves in response to economic, clinical, and political pressures, the role of EDs is evolving as well.

Because EDs charge higher prices for minor illness and injury care than other ambulatory care settings, ED care is frequently characterized as "the most expensive care there is." But this depiction ignores the many roles that EDs fill, and the statutory obligation of hospital EDs to provide care to all in need without regard for their ability to pay. To develop a more complete picture of how EDs contribute to our modern health care system, the Emergency Medicine Action Fund asked RAND to conduct this mixed-methods study.

At the outset of our effort, we reviewed recently published literature regarding ED use and used it to craft a conceptual model that depicts the various choices ED patients and providers make over the course of an episode of care. To quantify the importance of EDs as a major portal of entry to inpatient care, we analyzed four datasets compiled and maintained by the U.S. Department of Health and Human Services. Given a growing focus at the national and state levels on preventing non-urgent patients from seeking care in EDs, we analyzed data from the Community Tracking Study, a decade-long effort that describes changing patterns of health care utilization and delivery in 60 communities nationwide. To add context to the quantitative observations derived from these analyses, we conducted three focus groups with emergency medicine and hospitalist physicians, and interviewed 16 practicing primary care physicians who work in a variety of communities.

Key findings include the following:

- Between 2003 and 2009, inpatient admissions to U.S. hospitals grew at a slower rate than the population overall. However, nearly all of the growth in admissions was due to a 17 percent increase in unscheduled inpatient admissions from EDs. This growth in ED admissions more than offset a 10 percent decrease in admissions from doctors' offices and other outpatient settings. This pattern suggests that office-based physicians are directing to EDs some of the patients they previously admitted to the hospital.
- In addition to serving as an increasingly important portal of hospital admissions, EDs support primary care practices by performing complex diagnostic workups and handling overflow, after-hours, and weekend demand for care. Almost all of the physicians we interviewed—specialist and primary care alike—confirmed that office-based physicians increasingly rely on EDs to evaluate complex patients with potentially serious problems, rather than managing these patient themselves.
- As a result of these shifts in practice, emergency physicians are increasingly serving as the major decisionmaker for approximately half of all hospital admissions in the United States. This role has important financial implications, not only because admissions

generate the bulk of facility revenue for hospitals, but also because inpatient care accounts for 31 percent of national health care spending.

- Although the core role of EDs is to evaluate and stabilize seriously ill and injured patients, the vast majority of patients who seek care in an ED walk in the front door and leave the same way. Data from the Community Tracking Study indicate that most ambulatory patients do not use EDs for the sake of convenience. Rather, they seek care in EDs because they perceive no viable alternative exists, or because a health care provider sent them there.

- Medicare accounts for more inpatient admissions from EDs than any other payer. To gain insight into whether care coordination makes a difference in the likelihood of hospital admission from an ED, we compared ED admission rates among Medicare beneficiaries enrolled in a Medicare Choice plan versus beneficiaries enrolled in Medicare fee-for-service (FFS). We found no clear effect on inpatient admissions overall, or on a subset of admissions involving conditions that might be considered "judgment calls."

- Irrespective of the impact of care coordination, EDs may be playing a constructive role in constraining the growth of inpatient admissions. Although the number of non-elective ED admissions has increased substantially over the past decade, inpatient admissions of ED patients with "potentially preventable admissions" (as defined by the Agency for Healthcare Research and Quality) are flat over this time interval.

Our study indicates that: (1) EDs have become an important source of admissions for American hospitals; (2) EDs are being used with increasing frequency to conduct complex diagnostic workups of patients with worrisome symptoms; (3) Despite recent efforts to strengthen primary care, the principal reason patients visit EDs for non-emergent outpatient care is lack of timely options elsewhere; and (4) EDs may be playing a constructive role in preventing some hospital admissions, particularly those involving patients with an ambulatory care sensitive condition. Policymakers, third party payers, and the public should be aware of the various ways EDs meet the health care needs of the communities they serve and support the efforts of ED providers to more effectively integrate ED operations into both inpatient and outpatient care.

Acknowledgements

Numerous individuals and organizations provided source material or substantive assistance to this report. Our quantitative analysis used data from several sources, including the Agency for Healthcare Research and Quality, the Center for Studying Health Systems Change and the Inter-university Consortium for Political and Social Research and the National Center for Health Statistics at the Centers for Disease Control and Prevention (CDC). Several organizations allowed us to recruit from their memberships for focus groups. These include: the American College of Emergency Physicians (ACEP), the Society for Academic Emergency Medicine, The Patient Centered Primary Care Collaborative, and the Society for Hospital Medicine. Several individuals were particularly helpful to the recruiting effort: Susan Spradlin, Buck Beighley, and Peggy Brock (ACEP); Amy Gibson, Michelle Shaljian, Dr. Paul Grundy, Marci Nielsen, and Deborah Felsenthal (The Patient Centered Primary Care Collaborative), Dr. Joe Stubbs, former President of the American College of Physicians, and Dr. Todd Von Deak, Dr. Mark Williams, and Dr. Larry Wellikson (Society for Hospital Medicine). Finally, we are particularly grateful for the outstanding technical advice and analytical assistance we received from Ryan Mutter of the Agency for Healthcare Research and Quality, and the thoughtful comments and suggestions of Andrew Mulcahy and Lori Uscher-Pines of the RAND Corporation and Stephen R. Pitts of Emory University.

Abbreviations

ACEP	American College of Emergency Physicians
ACO	Accountable Care Organization
ACS	Ambulatory Care Sensitive
AHRQ	Agency for Healthcare Research and Quality
CCS	Clinical Classifications Software
CDC	Center for Disease Control and Prevention
CHIP	Children's Health Insurance Program
COPD	chronic obstructive pulmonary disease
CT	computerized tomographic
CTS	Community Tracking Study
ED	Emergency Department
EMAF	Emergency Medicine Action Fund
EMR	Electronic Medical Record
EMTALA	Emergency Medical Treatment and Labor Act
ER	Emergency Room
FFS	Fee-for-Service
GDP	Gross Domestic Product
HCUP	Healthcare Cost and Utilization Project
HMO	Health Maintenance Organization
ICD-9-CM	International Classification of Diseases, Ninth Revision, Clinical Modification
ICU	Intensive Care Unit
IT	Information Technology
NEDS	Nationwide Emergency Department Sample
NHDS	National Hospital Discharge Survey
NCHS	National Center for Health Statistics
NIS	Nationwide Inpatient Sample
PCP	Primary Care Physician
PPO	Preferred Provider Organization
PQI	Prevention Quality Indicators
SEDD	State Emergency Department Database
SID	State Inpatient Database

1. Introduction

This report examines the evolving role of hospital emergency departments (EDs) in the U.S. health care system. RAND conducted the study at the request of the Emergency Medicine Action Fund to develop a comprehensive picture of how EDs contribute to modern health care and to suggest how ED care might be more effectively, and more cost-effectively, integrated with community care.

Trends Affecting the Evolution of Hospital EDs

The hospital ED is a relatively recent phenomenon that emerged in the years following World War II (A. L. Kellermann & Martinez, 2011). Beginning in the early 1970s and accelerating through the 1980s and 1990s, ED staffing shifted from part-time coverage by community physicians, rotating house officers, or moonlighters to full-time, around-the-clock coverage by residency-trained, board-certified emergency physicians (IOM, 2007). The highly specialized knowledge and skills these doctors possess have allowed hospital EDs to dramatically expand their capability to diagnose and manage a wide range of problems, from resuscitating critically ill and injured children and adults to managing complex patients with chronic diseases such as HIV–AIDS, cancer, renal failure, and diabetes. The enhanced capability to manage complex and time-critical problems has also given ED staff more options to diagnose and manage problems without resorting to hospital admission.

Overall Growth in Health Care Spending.

The evolving role of EDs in America's health care system must be viewed against the backdrop of a seemingly relentless rise in the rate of health care cost growth. For most of the past 60 years, U.S. health care spending outgrew gross domestic product (GDP) by an average of 2–2.3 percentage points per year (Fuchs, 2012). In 1990, the United States spent 12 percent of GDP, roughly $724 billion, on health care. In 2010, health care devoured 17.9 percent of GDP, $2.6 trillion (Center for Medicare and Medicaid Services, 2012). Spending growth has slowed since 2009 (Davis, 2011), but experts debate whether this reflects changes in health care delivery or a sluggish recovery from the recession that began the previous year.

Health care has grown so expensive that it is threatening the viability of employer-sponsored health insurance (Kaiser Family Foundation, 2012) and the solvency of the Medicare program. (Ginsburg, 2008). States have less money for education and other important priorities (Pew Center on the States, 2012). Between 1999 and 2009, health care cost growth wiped out the income gains of middle class families (Auerbach & Kellermann, 2011).

Spending growth is the top concern of policymakers; however, despite the fact that hospital ED use has increased, the ED contribution to spending growth is small. ED care is widely characterized as the most expensive care there is, but the real issue for EDs—one misunderstood by policymakers—is not the cost of non-urgent use. Rather, it is the growing role that EDs play as gateways to inpatient treatment, which accounts for 31 percent of health care spending.

Growing Use of Hospital EDs

Between 2001 and 2008, use of hospital EDs grew at roughly twice the rate of population growth (Kharbanda et al., 2013). During the same period, hospitals closed about 198,000 beds. With more patients seeking care and fewer inpatient beds available for those who need one, EDs grew crowded with admitted patients who could not be transitioned to inpatient care. (Kellermann, 2006).

Practice intensity has also increased in EDs, in part because EDs are treating older and sicker patients, and in part because emergency physicians are bringing more sophisticated and costly technology, such as more aggressive use of computerized tomographic (CT) scanning and other diagnostic tests, to bear in managing their patients' problems. In 2012, Pitts and colleagues noted that "EDs have become a central staging area for acutely ill patients, for the use of diagnostic technology, and for decisions about hospital admission, all of which makes ED care increasingly complex" (Pitts, Pines, Handrigan, & Kellermann, 2012). The combined effects of steady growth of ED visits, more-intensive workups, and fewer inpatient beds have extended ED lengths of stay, dramatically increasing the number of patients in hospital EDs at any hour of the day (Pitts et al., 2012). The crowding that results compromises patient safety and can worsen patient outcomes (Bernstein et al., 2009).

The increase in practice intensity also generated higher charges. Although emergency medicine's contribution to aggregate physician charges in the United States is relatively small, a team of Harvard analysts determined that emergency medicine has boosted its Medicare charges relative to its 2002 baseline faster than almost every other specialty, ranking second only to radiation oncology (Alhassani, Chandra, & Chernew, 2012).

Basic issues of access are key determinants of ED use. EDs are the only place in the U.S. health care system where the poor cannot be turned away. As a result, they are disproportionately used by low-income and uninsured patients who cannot reliably get care in other settings. In fact, the 4 percent of doctors who staff America's EDs manage 28 percent of all acute care visits in the United States, half of all the acute care provided to Medicaid and Children's Health Insurance Program (CHIP) beneficiaries, and two-thirds of the acute care provided to the uninsured (Pitts, Carrier, Rich, & Kellermann, 2010).

The Rising Cost of ED Care

ED charges for treatment of adults have grown dramatically. Between 2001 and 2010, physician claims for higher-paid services, particularly level 5 visits (the highest level of severity in Medicare coding), grew from 27 percent to 48 percent of Medicare discharges (Office of Inspector General, 2012).

Politicians are fond of asserting that "emergency department care is the most expensive care there is." The numbers suggest otherwise. EDs provide 11 percent of all outpatient visits and are the portal of entry for roughly half of all hospital admissions (Pitts et al., 2010); however, they account for only 2–4 percent of total annual health care expenditures (American College of Emergency Physicians, 2012). Recently, the McKinsey Global Institute estimated that aggregate national spending on outpatient health care totaled about $850 billion in 2006 (McKinsey Global Institute, 2008). Of that, less than 10 percent ($75 billion) could be attributed to EDs, suggesting that aggregate spending for ED care is in line with its share of outpatient care delivery.

Studies of ED charges versus reimbursement have generated mixed results. Rates of reimbursement for pediatric ED visits decreased significantly from 1996 to 2003 (Hsia, MacIsaac, & Baker, 2008). Among adult patients, charges and associated payments for ED care have increased, due at least in part to the steady growth of ED visits (Pitts, Niska, Xu, & Burt, 2008).

Both inefficiencies in the health care system and legal requirements contribute to ED costs. Providers often feel obliged to repeat tests because they cannot get access to the patient's medical record. High levels of uncompensated care also figure prominently in ED costs. Because EDs are required under federal law to evaluate and stabilize all who present to the ED without regard for ability to pay, they serve as the "safety net of the safety net" for uninsured patients and Medicaid beneficiaries (Schuur & Venkatesh, 2012; Tang, Stein, Hsia, Maselli, & Gonzales, 2010). Nationwide, about 55 percent of emergency services are uncompensated (American College of Emergency Physicians, 2012).

Efforts to Discourage Non-Urgent Use of EDs

Cognizant of the high charges associated with ED visits, health plans and government are taking increasingly aggressive action to discourage non-urgent ED visits (Baker, 1994; Washington, Stevens, Shekelle, Henneman, & Brook, 2002). Arguing that such visits can be readily managed in less costly settings, policymakers and third-party payers have considered a variety of strategies to steer patients away from EDs and to deny payment for non-urgent ED visits (Cutler, 2010). Shifting ED patients to less expensive outpatient or office-based care is appealing in concept, but difficult to accomplish in practice (Florence, 2005). There is no standard definition of non-urgent care. In addition, it is notoriously difficult to determine at ER triage which patients are really sick and which are not (A. L. W. Kellermann, R. M., 2012). Raven and colleagues, analyzing data from the National Hospital Ambulatory Medical Care Survey-ED subsample, determined that many patients with the same presenting complaint as those who were felt to be inappropriate ED visitors were found to require immediate emergency care or hospital admission (Raven, Lowe, Maselli, & Hsia, 2013).

Timeliness also plays a role in ED use. Research teams that have asked patients why they sought treatment in EDs for non-urgent conditions found that the primary motivator is lack of options, not lack of judgment (J. Billings, Parikh, & Mijanovich, 2000; J. Billings, Parikh, N., Mijanovich, T.,, 2000; Delia & Cantor, 2009; Goodell, 2009; A. L. W. Kellermann, R. M., 2012; Taylor, 2006; Young, Wagner, Kellermann, Ellis, & Bouley, 1996)). Indeed, a major driver of ED use is lack of access to primary care. When Americans develop an acute health problem, they see their primary care provider less than half the time, especially when the symptoms involve a potentially serious problem, such as chest or abdominal pain, headache, shortness of breath, or other potentially serious problems (Pitts et al., 2010). A survey by the Centers for Disease Control and Prevention (CDC) conducted in 2011 showed that about 80 percent of adults who visited an ED did so because they lacked access to other providers. Nearly half reported "the doctor's office was not open" as the reason for their most recent ED visit (CDC, 2012).

EDs as Entry Points to Inpatient Care

Little thought has been given to the growing role that EDs play as gateways to inpatient treatment, which accounts for one-third of health care spending. Between 1993 and 2006, hospital admissions from the ED grew by 50 percent (from 11.5 million to 17.3 million). As a result, the share of inpatient stays that originated in the ED increased from 34 percent to 44 percent (Schuur & Venkatesh, 2012).

Although EDs are essential to hospital operations, many administrators consider their ED a "loss leader" (Hsia, Kellermann, & Shen, 2011; Simonet, 2009). This perception is due, in part, to the financial burden of uncompensated care that EDs are legally required to provide, and in part to accounting practices that attribute inpatient revenues to the admitting service, rather than the department where the admission originated (Institute of Medicine, 2007).

Recently, Smulowitz, Honigman and Landon (Smulowitz, Honigman, & Landon, 2013) proposed a novel framework that classifies ED visits into broad categories of severity and seeks to focus the attention of policymakers and health system managers on ED visits that present the most potential for improving outcomes while simultaneously reducing costs. The approach they devised suggests that the current focus on diverting low-acuity visits to less-costly sites of ambulatory care would not produce savings of the magnitude that could be achieved if EDs and their associated health systems focused on reducing preventable hospital admissions and, to a lesser extent, improving ED care of patients with what the authors term "intermediate or complex conditions." After outlining this framework, the authors proposed a variety of ways in which EDs might become more fully integrated into a health care delivery system that puts patients first.

The project described in this report was nearly finished when Smulowitz et al. published their paper; however, in many ways our study results have provided empirical support of their work.

Aims of the RAND Study

In a series of three reports published in 2006, the Institute of Medicine (IOM) examined the strengths, limitations, and future challenges of emergency care in the U.S. health system (Institute of Medicine, 2007). The IOM noted that tremendous progress has been made in the science of emergency medicine, the capabilities of emergency care providers, the development of emergency medical services (EMS), and the regionalization of trauma care. It also noted that hospital-based emergency care has grown so overburdened, it has reached "the breaking point" (Institute of Medicine, 2007).

With the exception of the IOM, few independent groups have examined the various roles that EDs play, the challenges they face, and the contributions they make to the functioning of our nation's health care system. This information gap makes it difficult to understand how EDs should be integrated into community-based care.

The overarching goal of our work was to help fill this information gap. Our study had five specific aims:

1. *Quantify and contrast the number and percentage of hospital admission decisions made by ED physicians compared with those of primary care physicians (PCPs) and other office-based specialists.* We hypothesized that the percentage of admissions entering the hospital through the ED has grown relative to the number of patients directly admitted from their physician's office.
2. *Quantify the proportion of non-elective admissions that enter hospitals through the ED versus direct admissions from physicians' offices and other primary care settings.* We hypothesized that the proportion of hospital admissions that is non-elective has increased and that this increase is being driven by admissions entering via the ED.[1]
3. *Determine the frequency and reasons why office-based physicians refer patients to the ED for evaluation and, if required, hospitalization, rather than directly admitting the patient themselves.* We hypothesized that office-based physicians are increasingly using the ED for evaluating and admitting non-elective patients.
4. *Determine ED admission rates by type of health care insurance for various sub-populations of interest.* We hypothesized that the number and rate of ED admissions (as a percentage of total ED visits by payer group) is growing more quickly among Medicare beneficiaries and privately insured patients than among Medicaid beneficiaries and the uninsured. Furthermore, we hypothesized that patients enrolled in a health plan that offers care coordination are less likely to be hospitalized than otherwise comparable patients who are covered by a fee-for-service (FFS) plan.
5. *Determine if EDs are playing a role in reducing preventable hospital admissions and readmissions of patients with ambulatory care sensitive (ACS) conditions* (e.g., asthma,

---

[1] Non-elective admissions are urgent/emergent hospitalizations dictated by the patient's medical condition and their treating physician's determination that hospitalization is required to address the problem. Generally speaking, they cannot be postponed. Elective admissions are chosen by the patient or their physician for reasons that are perceived to be beneficial to the patient, but are not urgent.

diabetes, heart failure, other chronic health conditions). We hypothesized that although ED use by patients with ACS conditions is growing, the number of hospitalizations involving these same clinical conditions is either flat or rising at a slower rate. If true, this may indicate that EDs are playing a constructive role in reducing preventable hospital admissions.

Organization of This Report

The discussion that follows is organized as follows. We describe our conceptual model of ED use (Chapter Two), methods (Chapter Three), findings (Chapter Four), and their implications (Chapter Five). We conclude by drawing conclusions for policy and practice (Chapter Six).

2. Conceptual Model of ED Use

To conceptualize the various ways a patient with a new health problem or worsening chronic condition weighs options for care and navigates the health care system, we developed a logic model (see Figure 2.1). It draws on previous logic models built around patient decisionmaking and the operation of hospital EDs (Asplin et al., 2003 2012; Pitts et al., 2010; Uscher-Pines, Pines, Kellermann, Gillen, & Mehrotra, 2013). Specifically, we linked the Uscher-Pines model of patient choice with the Asplin model of ED input-throughput-output to determine the various options available to a typical patient. We have added a referral component, since primary care physicians can either directly admit an ill patient to the hospital or refer them to a nearby ED. On occasion, urgent care clinics and retail clinics also refer patients to the ED.

Figure 2.1. Conceptual Model for ED Use

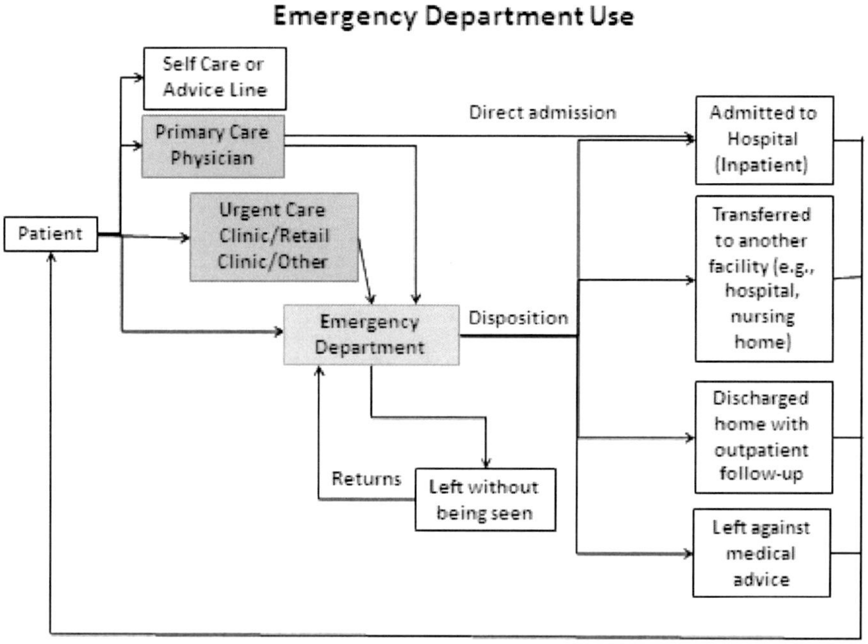

Emergency Department Use

Figure 2.1 highlights a patient's possible decision pathways regarding ED use. In the discussion below, we describe clinical decision points on the pathway. They include: (1) patient chooses to seek medical care from various options, including the ED; (2) primary care physician chooses to either directly admit a patient or refer to the ED; and (3) emergency physician determines the patient's disposition from an array of options. At the end of the process, a patient may start the cycle over again by returning to his/her primary care provider or by making a repeat visit to the ED.

7

When a patient develops a potentially serious, worrisome, or physically uncomfortable problem, such as shortness of breath or chest pain, he or she faces a series of choices (Morgan et al., 2012). These include: (1) ignore the problem and hope it gets better; (2) self-medicate; (3) seek treatment from a primary care provider (MD, NP, other)/medical home (Flottemesch, Anderson, Solberg, Fontaine, & Asche, 2012); (4) seek treatment in a retail clinic or urgent care center (or other); and (5) seek treatment in an ED. We present these options in Figure 2.2, building on a patient choice model developed by Uscher-Pines and colleagues (Uscher-Pines et al., 2013).

Figure 2.2. Health Care Options for Patients

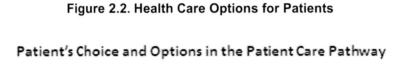

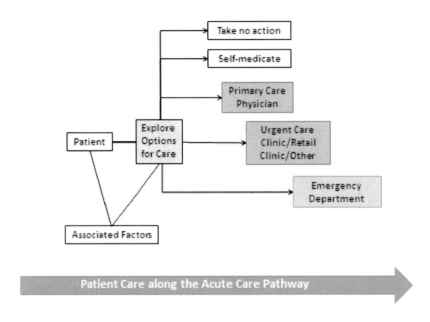

In a case of sudden or severe illness or serious injury, the decision to seek care is clear-cut. The only question is which source of care to choose, and whether to seek transport by ambulance or private vehicle. In other situations, however, the decision is less clear-cut. In their analysis, Uscher-Pines and her colleagues (Uscher-Pines et al., 2013) examined how patients with less serious illnesses or injuries weigh the pros and cons of various options for care, and the factors they consider in making their choice. Uscher-Pines' analysis was informed by a conceptual model (Figure 2.3).

Figure 2.3. Causal Pathway Factors and Associated Factors for Exploring Options of Care

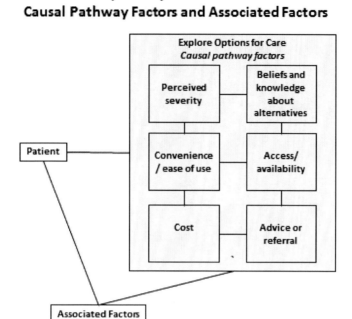

Source: Uscher-Pines et al., 2013.

In Uscher-Pines' view, patients' decisions to seek a specific source of care may be influenced by both causal and associated factors. Causal factors act as independent predictors of a specific source of care (Uscher-Pines et al., 2013); that is, there is a direct link between the factor and the choice to be made. Examples of causal factors include patients' perception of the severity of their symptoms (Johnson et al., 2012), their beliefs and knowledge of various care alternatives, the availability of health care and their ability to access it (Taylor, 2012), cost (Devries, Li, & Oza, 2013; Volpp, Loewenstein, & Asch, 2012), advice or referral (Kumar & Klein, 2012), and convenience or ease of use.

Associated factors also influence where patients choose to receive care; however, this influence is via one or more pathways (Begley, Behan, & Seo, 2010; Uscher-Pines et al., 2013). Associated factors include demographic factors such as patient age, sex, and race; income, education, and occupation (Rasch, Gulley, & Chan, 2012); health insurance (Community Memorial Hospital, 2012; Glendenning-Napoli, Dowling, Pulvino, Baillargeon, & Raimer, 2012; Simonet, 2009); social support; health status; personality; and previous health care experience and cultural or community norms regarding care seeking (Uscher-Pines et al. 2012). For example, patients of a certain age or occupation may be more likely to seek a certain source of care, but a patient's choice is not directly affected by the fact that he/she belongs to that age or occupation group.

9

An individual may decide to seek primary care instead of going to an ED. However, the patient may end up in an ED anyway, for multiple reasons (Young et al., 1996):

- The patient cannot contact a PCP and decides that the only alternative is an ED.
- The patient gets a pre-recorded message on the PCP's phone line (e.g., "if this is an emergency, please hang up and dial 911").
- The PCP or staff answer the phone but cannot accommodate the patient within a reasonable time frame (e.g., schedule full, call received at the end of the workday or the end of the work week).
- The PCP or staff conclude, based on the caller's description of symptoms, that ED care is warranted.
- The PCP sees the patient and determines that immediate ED referral or admission is warranted.
- Patient needs one or more diagnostic tests that are not available in the PCP's office but can be obtained in an ED (e.g., CT scan).
- The PCP declines to see the patient because he or she is uninsured or not covered by a type of insurance (e.g., Medicaid) that is attractive to the provider. (MetroHealth Medical Center, 2012; Weber, Showstack, Hunt, Colby, & Callaham, 2005; Weber et al., 2008). In this instance, the provider or staff may advise the patient to seek care in an ED, where the Emergency Medical Treatment and Labor Act (EMTALA) applies (Kellerman, 1994). Unlike doctors' offices and ambulatory care practices, hospital-based EDs are legally mandated under EMTALA to evaluate and, if necessary, stabilize all patients who present for care, regardless of their ability to pay.

Instead of seeing their PCP, the patient may go to a retail clinic or urgent care center (McKinlay & Marceau, 2012; Mehrotra & Lave, 2012; Mehrotra, Wang, Lave, Adams, & McGlynn, 2008; Ranseen TA, 1983; Reid et al., 2012; Snell, Jones, & Yoder, 1987; Wang, Ryan, McGlynn, & Mehrotra, 2010). Once there, the patient may be referred to an ED for the same reasons described above. In addition, because retail clinics and urgent care centers generally cannot admit patients to the hospital (Merritt, Naamon, & Morris, 2000), they have no choice but to refer seriously ill or injured cases to an ED.

PCPs generally have the option to admit an ill patient to the hospital themselves (i.e., a "direct admit"), or to refer the patient to an ED for evaluation and an independent decision. Reasons to favor the latter strategy include the following:

- Provider lacks admitting privileges at the patient's preferred hospital
- Provider has insufficient time to complete the admission process (e.g., admission often requires pulling paperwork together, making one or more calls to arrange for a bed, and writing admitting orders)
- The patient is unstable
- ED evaluation is needed to determine the need for admission (e.g., abdominal pain in an elderly patient, acute chest discomfort in a middle-aged man or woman).

Once a patient arrives at an ED, his or her care may follow one of several different paths. The most widely accepted depiction of this process is Asplin's Input-Throughput-Output Model (Asplin et al., 2003), depicted in Figure 2.4.

Figure 2.4. Conceptual Model for Emergency Department Care

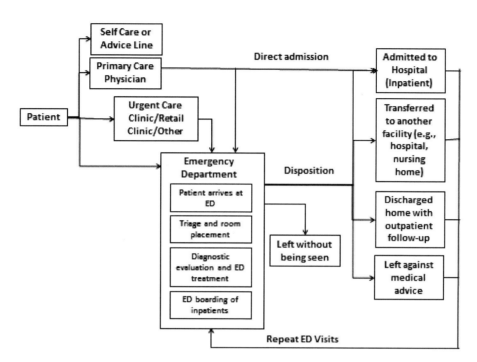

Once the ED evaluation is completed, the treating emergency physician has several options. These include:

- Admit the patient to the hospital, including hospital admissions to an intensive care unit, step-down unit, or a regular inpatient bed (McNeeley, Gunn, & Robinson, 2013; O'Mahony et al., 2013; Pines, Mutter, & Zocchi, 2013)
- Transfer the patient to another facility, including transfer to another acute care hospital (this may be done for clinical, personal, or economic reasons, such as the hospital is "in-network" versus "out-of-network") or transfer to a skilled nursing facility
- Discharge home with outpatient follow-up
- Patient leaves the ED against medical advice.

An additional option not shown in Figure 2.4 is to place the patient in an ED-based observation unit or inpatient unit on "observation status" for a protracted period of time to clarify their condition.

The complex interplay of patient, PCP, and ED physician considerations determines the ultimate path of each episode of care. The aggregate impact of these decisions contributes to the

11

annual cost of acute care in the United States. Because many ED encounters result in hospital admission, they have fiscal implications beyond the ED stay itself, since an average inpatient admission costs ten times more than an ED visit. In addition, inpatient admissions are the largest single source of health care spending in the United States, representing almost one third of total annual spending (Martin, Lassman, Washington, Catlin, & the National Health Expenditure Accounts Team, 2012).

3. Methods

Our project is primarily a quantitative analysis, supplemented by qualitative focus groups and interviews to provide context and potential explanations for our main observations. We obtained quantitative data from five nationally representative surveys (Owens et al., 2010). We obtained qualitative data from focus group discussions with ED physicians and hospitalists, and from individual interviews with primary care providers.

Quantitative Data Sources

Our data were drawn from five public-access data sets:

1. The National Hospital Discharge Survey (NHDS)

The NHDS, conducted annually by the CDC's National Center for Health Statistics (NCHS), covers discharges from non-institutional hospitals located in the 50 States and the District of Columbia.[2] The original sampling frame consisted of hospitals contained in the April 1987 *Hospital Market Database* from SMG Marketing Group, Inc. (Graves, 1995). This database is updated every three years to allow for hospital openings and closures, and to capture changes in survey eligibility. The NHDS uses a modified, three-stage sampling design.[3] In Stage 1, hospitals or geographic areas, such as counties, groups of counties, or metropolitan statistical areas, are selected. In Stage 2, additional hospitals are drawn from within sampled geographic areas. In Stage 3, discharges are sampled from selected hospitals. Beginning in 2008, the number of surveyed hospitals was reduced due to funding limitations.

The NHDS data provide detailed information on the type of admission (e.g., emergency, urgent, elective, or newborn) as well as the source of admission (e.g., physician referral, clinical referral, HMO referral, transfer [by specific types], emergency room). The NHDS also includes demographic data, allowing analysts to do subgroup and temporal comparisons while controlling for age, gender, and race as well as geographic region and type of hospital ownership.

We rely on NHDS data from 2003–2009 for two reasons. First, the rate of missing values in the type of admission and source of admission variables is above 20 percent in 2001 and 2002, rendering inferences unreliable. Second, guidance from the Centers for Medicare & Medicaid Services for coding source of admission changed in 2010, so that comparisons with earlier years

---

[2] This excludes Federal, military, and Veteran's Affairs hospitals. It also excludes long-stay hospitals (hospitals with an average length of stay for all patients of greater than 30 days).

[3] The current sampling design was instituted in 1988. Prior to 1988, the NHDS used a two-stage design. For a detailed description, see (Dennison & Pokras, 2000).

are not reliable.[4] We report the estimates for 2001, 2002, and 2010 in Appendix A (Tables A.1–A.7)[5] but do not include them in our figures. Sample sizes for each year of data are contained in Table 3.1.

Table 3.1. National Hospital Discharge Survey Sample Sizes, 2001–2010

Year	# Reporting Hospitals	Unweighted Response Rate (%)	# Total Discharges	# Non-newborn Discharges
2001	448	94%	330,210	293,800
2002	445	94%	327,254	292,059
2003	426	89%	319,530	285,436
2004	439	92%	370,785	331,222
2005	444	94%	375,372	335,670
2006	438	92%	376,328	336,302
2007	422	88%	365,648	325,615
2008	207	87%	165,630	149,396
2009	205	86%	162,151	146,501
2010	203	86%	151,551	137,459

2. Healthcare Cost and Utilization Project (HCUP) Nationwide Inpatient Sample (NIS)

Collected annually by the Agency for Healthcare Research and Quality (AHRQ), the NIS is the largest nationally representative all-payer inpatient care database publicly available in the United States. The NIS contains data on 5–8 million inpatient stays yearly from about 1,000 community hospitals from 1988 to 2010. It provides detailed information on the source of admission (e.g., ED vs. other sources) and insurance (payer) type for each inpatient stay (e.g., Medicare, Medicare Advantage, Medicaid, PPO, HMO, self-pay), as well as admission type (e.g., emergency, urgent, elective). The NIS also includes demographic and health status data, allowing analysts to do subgroup and temporal comparisons while controlling for age, underlying health status, and illness severity.

3. HCUP Nationwide Emergency Department Sample (NEDS)

The NEDS is the largest all-payer ED database that is publicly available in the United States. As of 2009, NEDS contains information on nearly 29 million ED visits to 964 hospitals that approximate a 20 percent stratified sample of U.S. hospital-based EDs. The NEDS is constructed out of two other HCUP files, the State Inpatient Database (SID) and State Emergency Department Database (SEDD) files. In states that share their data with AHRQ, the SEDD captures the universe of ED encounters in acute care hospitals that result in any disposition *other*

---

[4] Anjali Talwalkar (NCHS, personal communication).

[5] Appendix material for this report is available online at http://www.rand.org/pubs/research_reports/RR280.html

than admission to the same hospital. In these same states, the SID captures the universe of inpatient admissions to acute care hospitals in a state, including those that began in the ED. All of the ED encounters in states that submit to SID and SEDD form the sampling frame of the NEDS.

To build the NEDS, AHRQ sampled EDs, capturing all of the encounters in each sampled ED. The NEDS was constructed using records from both the HCUP SEDD and the SID. The NEDS includes records for ED visits that resulted in an admission (from the SID) and also includes ED visits that did not result in admission (e.g., treated and released, transferred to another hospital, transferred to another type of health facility, left against medical advice, died in ED) (from the SEDD). The NEDS is built using a 20 percent stratified sample of hospital-based EDs. All visits within the sample of selected EDs are included. So, if a hospital-based ED is selected for the NEDS sample, then all of the ED admissions from the SID and all of the ED visits from the SEDD are included in the NEDS.

The NEDS is composed of more than 100 variables, including: International Classification of Diseases, Ninth Revision, Clinical Modification (ICD-9-CM) diagnoses, CPT-4 procedures, discharge status from the ED, patient demographics (e.g., gender, age, urban-rural designation of residence, national quartile of median household income for patient's ZIP Code), and expected payment source (e.g., Medicare, Medicaid, private insurance, self-pay). The NEDS is weighted to yield national estimates of ED encounters.

4. Community Tracking Study (CTS) Household Survey and Health Tracking Household Surveys

The CTS and Health Tracking Household surveys are nationally representative household surveys that track changes in health care access and utilization, including ED visits from 1996–2010. The CTS was sponsored by the Robert Wood Johnson Foundation. Six waves of surveys were conducted: 1996–97, 1998–99, 2000–01, 2003, 2007, and 2010. (Early waves of this survey are referred to as CTS Household Surveys, but the 2007 and 2010 waves are referred to as the Health Tracking Household Surveys.) The 2003 CTS survey collected data on whether each ED visit resulted in a hospital stay, whether the patient contacted their personal physician before coming to the ED, and whether the patient's ED visit was recommended by his/her physician. Some survey questions differed from year to year, limiting our ability to track every relevant response over the CTS' full time span. The 2010 Health Tracking Household survey collected data on whether patients had a usual source of care, whether their health care provider's office has hours at night or on the weekends, and how difficult it is to contact a health care provider after their regular hours in case of urgent medical needs.

5. CTS Physician Survey and the Health System Change (HSC) Health Tracking Physician Study

The CTS Physician Survey was conducted in 1996–97, 1998–99, 2000–01, and 2004–05. Each of the first three surveys included responses from approximately 12,000 physicians; the fourth included more than 6,600 physicians. Data collection focused primarily on physicians practicing in 60 randomly selected U.S. communities, allowing analyses to be conducted at both the national and community level. In 2008, the CTS Physician Survey was replaced by the HSC Health Tracking Physician Survey, which gathered information from a nationally representative sample of more than 4,700 physicians and was conducted by mail by Westat (Center for Studying Health System Change, 2013).

Both the CTS physician surveys and the HSC 2008 Health Tracking Physician Survey cover a wide variety of physician and practice dimensions, from basic physician demographic information, practice organization, and career satisfaction to insurance acceptance, compensation arrangements, information technology use, and provision of charity care. The 2008 Health Tracking Physician Survey also included questions on care management, quality reporting, care coordination, malpractice concerns, ownership of hospitals and medical equipment, and greater detail on use of information technology. For this aspect of our analysis, we used data from both the 2004–05 CTS Physician Survey and the 2008 Health Tracking Physician Study. Both survey years included data on whether physicians were unable to obtain non-emergency hospital admissions for patients. Additionally, the 2004–05 CTS Physician Survey asked follow-up questions of all physicians who reported they were unable to obtain non-emergency hospital admissions for their patients in the past 12 months.

To generate insight into the challenges that PCPs face in admitting non-elective patients from their offices without sending them to an ED, we examined responses to the following physician questions from two waves of the CTS survey:

> Question: "During the last 12 months, were you unable to obtain any of the following services for your patients when you thought they were medically necessary? How about non-emergency hospital admissions?" (Source: Community Tracking Study 2004–05 Physician Survey)

> Question: "During the last 12 months, were you unable to obtain the following services for your patients when you thought they were medically necessary? How about non-emergency hospital admissions?" (Source: 2008 Health Tracking Physician Study)

To understand why responding physicians had difficulty, the 2004–05 version of the CTS Physician Survey asked a series of follow-up questions of all physicians who reported they were unable to obtain non-emergency hospital admissions for patients in past 12 months. The follow-up questions were only directed to PCPs, defined by the survey as general internal medicine and pediatrics, plus specialists in adolescent medicine, geriatric medicine, psychiatry, and obstetrics/gynecology.

> Question: "For each one (listed below), tell me whether it is a very important, moderately important, not very important, or not at all important reason for your being unable to obtain non-emergency hospital admissions.
>
> - There aren't enough qualified service providers or facilities in my area.
> - Health plan networks and administrative barriers limit patient access.

- Patients lack health insurance or have inadequate insurance coverage."
  (Source: Community Tracking Study 2004–05 Physician Survey)

To examine ED use from the patient's perspective, we used data from the 2003 CTS Household Study. This was the only edition of the CTS survey that collected detailed data on the number of times an individual sought medical care from an ED and related questions such as whether the patient attempted to contact his/her personal physician before seeking care in an ED, whether the patient's ED visit was recommended by his/her physician or a member of the physician's staff, whether alternatives to an ED were available, and whether the patient's ED visit resulted in a hospital inpatient stay.

Analytical Approach

Aim 1: Quantify and contrast the number and percentage of admission decisions made by ED physicians compared with those of other specialists and primary care physicians.
Aim 2: Quantify the proportion of non-elective admissions that enter hospitals through the ED versus direct admissions from a physician's office or other primary care settings.

To address aims 1 and 2, we carried out bivariate analyses of two variables in the NHDS, Type and Source of Admission (both available from 2001, although the amount of missing data was problematic until 2003). The available categories for Type of Admission included Emergency, Urgent, Elective, Newborn, and Not Available. In our analyses, we excluded newborn admissions and combined Emergency and Urgent into Non-Elective admission. The available categories for Source of Admission included Physician referral, Clinical referral, HMO referral, Transfer from a hospital, Transfer from a skilled nursing facility, Transfer from other health facility, Emergency room, Court/law enforcement, Other, and Not available. We combined the three transfers codes, Court/law enforcement, and Other into a single overall "Other" category. We added the very small share of HMO referrals to this group due to the uncertainty in coding. We also combined the Physician and Clinical referrals into a single category. Physician referrals account for more than 90 percent of all referrals in the NHDS.

The weighted proportion of non-newborn records in the NHDS that are coded "Not Available" for the source and type of admission decreases from 13 percent for both variables in 2003 to 3 percent and 6 percent in 2009, respectively. To address the problem of missing data, we adopted two different strategies. First, we imputed missing data under the assumption that missing data followed the same distribution as the (weighted) non-missing data within a year/region/sex/age group cell, e.g., using the distribution of non-missing values for the categorical variable for the admission source in 2004, for females aged 45–64 in the Northeast to correct the missing values for the admission source in the same group. We implemented this approach using single (conditional mean) imputation. Second, as any approach to imputation relies on assumptions, we also present estimates without imputation and include the missing value in a separate category termed "missing" (see Appendix A Tables A.5 and A.6, available online). All figures and tables in the main text show weighted estimates for non-newborn discharges for which missing values have been imputed.

We calculated standard errors using methods recommended by the CDC's NCHS. Because the NHDS does not include survey design variables, NCHS recommends that standard errors for frequencies be calculated using the formula

$$SE(X) = \left(\sqrt{a + b/X}\right) * X,$$

while standard errors for percentages were obtained using the formula

$$SE(p) = \left(\sqrt{\frac{b*(1-p)}{(p*X)}}\right) * p,$$

where p is the percentage of interest, and X is the denominator on which the percentage is based. The parameters a and b are provided by the NCHS in the documentation accompanying each dataset. Because the NCHS does not provide parameter values for subgroup analysis, we use values for the first-listed diagnosis. This procedure is recommended by NCHS staff and assumes the absence of clustering. In the main results section that follows, all of the figures and tables incorporate imputed data. Non-imputed data for the main tables are provided in Appendix A (Tables A.5 and A.6, available online), along with standard error tables (Appendix Table A.7, available online). To visually depict the impact of imputing, we provide two versions of key figures, so a reader can see how imputing missing data influences the shape of the graphs. Although there is some evidence that missing data, particularly in the earlier part of the decade, were not randomly distributed, we feel that imputing produces a more representative picture of the totality of hospital admissions than the alternative, which is to enumerate the "missing" cases in their own category.

Because these analyses involved very large samples, all but the smallest differences are statistically significant. For the sake of clarity and simplicity, we do not report statistical testing.

Aim 3: Determine the frequency and reasons why office-based physicians refer patients to the ED for evaluation and if required, hospitalization, rather than directly admitting the patient themselves.

To investigate the extent to which office-based physicians rely on EDs to help manage their patients, we used data from the CTS Physician Survey to estimate the proportion of physicians that reported being unable to obtain a non-emergency hospital admission for their patients.

We also explored why patients self-refer to the ED through two different analyses. First, we used data from the CTS Household Study data to assess the number of times per year that different individuals seek care from EDs. Additionally, using data from the 2003 CTS Household survey, we analyzed how often patients attempted to contact their personal physician before seeking care in an ED, whether the patient's ED visit was recommended by his/her physician or a member of the physician's staff, whether other alternatives to ED care were available, and whether the ED visit resulted in a hospital stay. We supplemented both analyses with qualitative information collected through our individual semi-structured interviews with PCPs, which are described in greater detail below.

Aim 4: Determine ED admission rates by type of health care insurance for various sub-populations of interest.

To examine how type of health insurance influences the nature and rate of ED admissions, we analyzed data from the HCUP NIS. First, we descriptively analyzed the frequency of ED and non-ED admissions by primary payer: Medicare, Medicaid, private (commercial insurance), and uninsured. Next, we identified changes in the number of unscheduled ED admissions by primary payer over time.

To give our team a preliminary look at whether or not health plans that offer care coordination make it easier for emergency physicians to discharge borderline cases rather than admit them to the hospital, colleagues at the AHRQ graciously agreed to run a special analysis of the SEDD file, limited to 20 states that provide coverage codes that allowed AHRQ's analysts to distinguish patients covered by a Medicare Advantage Plan versus Medicare FFS (Mutter R., personal communication) The dependent variable was defined as 1 if the patient was admitted to the hospital and 0 otherwise. The 20 states, designated by postal codes, were: AZ, CA, CT, FL, GA, HI, IA, KS, KY, MA, MD, MN, NJ, NV, NY, OH, RI, SD, TN, and WI.

To control for potentially confounding variables, the AHRQ team built logistic regression models that considered the potentially confounding effects of gender, age, and comorbidity, using Elixhauser comorbidity software variables (Elixhauser, Steiner, Whittington, et al., 1998). They also controlled for hospital location (urban versus rural), hospital teaching status (teaching versus nonteaching) and hospital ownership (private for profit, private non-profit, or public ownership). After examining the overall effect of Medicare Advantage on the probability of ED admission, they repeated the analysis after restricting it to certain ACS conditions included in the Clinical Classifications Software (CCS) system, a disease categorization scheme that collapses the ICD-9-CM diagnosis codes into 260 mutually exclusive, clinically meaningful categories (Healthcare Cost and Utilization Project, undated). For this analysis, the AHRQ team restricted their regression model to CCS categories 122 (pneumonia), 108 (congestive heart failure), 127 (chronic obstructive pulmonary disease, COPD), 102 (nonspecific chest pain), 237 (complications of a device, graft, or implant), 197 (skin and subcutaneous infection), 159 (urinary tract infection), and 55 (fluid and electrolyte disorders), because these diagnoses sometimes involve "judgment" calls regarding whether a fragile patient can be safely discharged home. If care coordination gives physicians a greater sense of security regarding discharging such cases, we might see lower rates of admission for these conditions among Medicare Advantage patients.

Aim 5: Quantify what role, if any, EDs play in reducing preventable hospital admissions and readmissions, particularly for patients with ambulatory care sensitive conditions.

To achieve this aim, we used data from the HCUP NEDS and NIS datasets. To estimate the number of hospital of admissions involving various ACS (Parmigiani et al., 2007) conditions, used by the AHRQ as "Prevention Quality Indicators" (PQI) to determine potentially preventable hospital admissions, we used software provided by AHRQ to calculate the annual frequency of PQI-related hospital admissions from EDs and other sources in the NIS (AHRQ, 2013). PQIs capture a range of important, treatable problems, such as diabetes complications, congestive heart failure, asthma, bacterial pneumonia, urinary tract infections, and other treatable conditions, into three broad indicators of prevention-related quality: Acute PQIs, Chronic PQIs, and an Overall PQI Score.

To determine trends of ED versus non-ED admissions related to PQIs, we needed some measure of rates of ED visits and analogous ED-related hospital admissions for each PQI diagnosis. Unfortunately, PQIs are only assigned to hospital admissions. To circumvent this obstacle, we used the Clinical Classifications Software (CCS) system, described in the previous paragraph (Healthcare Cost and Utilization Project, undated). Because CCS codes are available in the NEDS, we used this dataset to identify the percentage of ED visits and admissions by primary and secondary CCS categories that were admitted to the same hospital during 2006 and 2009. For our analysis, we chose CCS categories that corresponded well with a PQI (e.g., PQI conditions "diabetes short term complication" and "diabetes uncontrolled" were aligned with CCS code for "diabetes mellitus with complications'). This allowed us to make a rough approximation of whether changing numbers of ED admissions related to PQIs are being driven by changing numbers of ED visits related to a particular CCS, changing rates of admission for that condition, or both.

Table 3.2. Summary of Quantitative Data Sources, by Project Aim

Aim	Data Source	Key Variables	Years Analyzed
1 & 2	CDC's National Hospital Discharge Survey (NHDS)	Admission type (elective vs. non-elective) Source of admission	2003–2009
3	Community Tracking Study (CTS) Household Survey	Disposition of ED visit Source of ED visit (e.g., physician referral)	1996–97, 1998–99, 2000–01, 2003, 2007
	Community Tracking Study (CTS) Physician Survey and the Health Tacking Physician Study	Non-emergency hospital admissions	2004–05, 2008
4	HCUP Nationwide Inpatient Sample (NIS)	Source of admission Payer type	1993–2009

20

Aim	Data Source	Key Variables	Years Analyzed
5	HCUP Nationwide Emergency Department Sample (NEDS)	Disposition of ED visit ICD-9 CM Diagnosis	2006–2009
	HCUP Nationwide Inpatient Sample (NIS)	CPT codes ICD-9 CM procedures	1988–2009

Qualitative Data Sources

While the quantitative data are useful for identifying who, where, and when, they can rarely explain "why." To provide context for our quantitative analysis, we concurrently conducted three focus groups with ED physicians and hospitalists, and a series of individual interviews with practicing PCPs. The framework for the focus groups and interviews was crafted to explore potential explanations for the observations we anticipated would come from our quantitative analysis of the federal datasets. In practice, our focus groups and interviews were conducted after the initial data analysis for Aims 1 and 2 and in parallel with the data analyses we performed to address Aims 3 through 5. For this reason, our focus group guides and semi-structured interview instrument were structured to explore the same issues addressed in our specific aims. The focus group discussion guides and interview instrument can be found in Appendix B (available online).

Emergency Physician Focus Groups

We conducted two focus groups at the American College of Emergency Physicians (ACEP) Scientific Assembly in Denver, Colorado, on October 10, 2012. This annual meeting of the organization attracts over 5,000 emergency physicians from across the United States as well as from several international locations. We recruited participants by email distributed to ACEP's listserv of emergency physicians registered to attend the conference. Thirty participants and ten alternates were selected from an initial sign-up list of 158 respondents who completed an online survey about their years in practice, organizational affiliation, and practice environment. Participants were chosen to capture a wide representation of practice settings (see Appendix B, Table B.1, available online). To encourage participation and compensate discussants for their time, each participating provider received a $150 stipend.

Our moderators used a discussion guide that provided stimulus questions to engage each group in discussing four domains that were highly relevant to our analysis: (1) factors considered in admission decisions, (2) factors that lead PCPs to refer patients to the ED, (3) factors that contribute to "preventable" hospitalizations and repeat ED visits, and (4) discussant thoughts about how EDs influence health care costs. We also gave both ED focus groups an opportunity to raise other issues of concern to them (Appendix B, available online).

Hospital Physician Focus Group

To ascertain the perspective of practicing hospitalists, we recruited participants with the assistance of the Society for Hospital Medicine, a professional medical society that represents more than 10,000 of the 30,000 practicing hospitalists in the United States. Seven participants responded who completed an online survey about their years in practice, organizational affiliation, and practice environment (see Appendix B, Table B.2, available online). To encourage participation and compensate discussants for their time, each participating provider received a $150 stipend.

Using a combination of multiple choice poll questions and a semi-structured focus group protocol, we conducted a web-based focus group using PowerPoint slides and a teleconference line. Online focus groups have many benefits, including their relatively low cost and easier access to a broad range of potential participants (Gaiser, 2008). We asked hospitalist providers about a number of issues, including factors that impacted their admission decisions, their experiences with primary care provider referrals, factors associated with preventable ED visits, and opinions about the ED's role in increasing costs of health care (see Appendix B, available online).

All three focus groups were recorded and notes were taken by a trained research assistant. Each group lasted 1.5 hours. At least two members of the study team were involved in each focus group discussion. After each session, the focus group leaders and interviewers reviewed their notes and summarized and enumerated important themes. These were subsequently discussed with the project leaders to establish areas in which themes converged.

Individual Interviews with Primary Care Providers

To ascertain the perspective of primary care providers, we initially sought to recruit participants for a fourth focus group. We sought the assistance of the Patient-Centered Primary Care Collaborative, an organization dedicated to advancing primary care and patient-centered medical homes. Because we could not find a suitable time when a sufficient number of primary care providers could participate in a focus group, we opted to schedule individual interviews at the most convenient time for each provider. Individual interviews allowed us to better accommodate each provider's schedule and shorten the time requirement for each provider from 1.5 hours to 30 minutes. To compensate discussants for their time, each participating provider received a $75 stipend. We conducted interviews with sixteen physicians (see Appendix B, Table B.3, available online).

Using a semi-structured interview protocol, modeled after the focus group guides we used with emergency physicians and hospitalists, we asked participating PCPs their views and experiences related to a number of issues, including their experiences with ED referrals, factors that impacted their ED referrals, hospital admission decisions, factors that impacted their hospital admission decisions, opinions about the ED's role in health care costs, and the role that EDs play in helping them care for their patients. The interview instrument is included in Appendix B, available online.

Interview notes were taken by a trained research assistant. Each interview lasted approximately 30 minutes.

Review of Qualitative Data

We reviewed the interview notes from each focus group and summarized notes across groups to identify themes. Themes examined include inpatient admission decisions, ED referrals from primary care providers, preventable ED visits and readmissions, and the ED's impact on health care costs. Because the participants were drawn from convenience samples, our analysis focused on broad themes, and we did not apply the full range of methodological checks associated with formal qualitative research. Thus, we offer the output of this process with caveats regarding its representativeness to the national pool of practitioners. For this reason, we report only broad findings. Those who wish to review the interview instruments or summary notes of the focus groups and interviews can find them in Appendix B, available online.

4. Findings

In this chapter, we present the results of our quantitative analyses, and describe the major themes that emerged from our focus groups and individual interviews.[6] Our presentation of findings generally tracks the order of our study aims, but in this section we use specific questions to focus attention on individual aspects of our results.

What are the most important sources of inpatient admissions and how have they changed?

1. Between 2003 and 2009, the U.S. population grew at a rate of about 5.7 percent, from 290.8 million in 2003 to 307.4 million in 2009 (U.S. Census Bureau, 2012). During the same period, total inpatient admissions (elective and non-elective) grew at a rate of 4 percent, from roughly 34.7 million to 36.1 million.[7] ED admissions, which grew at a rate of about 17 percent, accounted for nearly all of this growth (Figure 4.1). This more than offset a 1.6 million decrease in direct admissions from physician's offices and clinics (from 15.6 to 14 million, a relative decline of 10 percent). Admissions from other sources, such as inter-facility transfers, rose only slightly and from a much smaller base. As a result, they made only a modest contribution to overall growth of hospital admissions.

---

[6] A more detailed version of the qualitative results is included in our online appendix, with representative quotes.

[7] The NIS data were fairly similar to the NHDS data reported. In 2003, there were 34.8 million total inpatient admissions in the NIS data (as compared to 34.7 million in the NHDS data). In 2009, there were 35.9 million total inpatient admissions in the NIS data (as compared to 36.1 million in the NHDS data). Additionally, the ED admissions data were similar between the NIS and the NHDS. ED admissions increased from 16.7 million in 2003 to 18.2 million in 2009 in the NIS data (as compared to 16.2 to 18.9 million in the NHDS).

Figure 4.1. Inpatient Admissions, by Source, 2003–2009

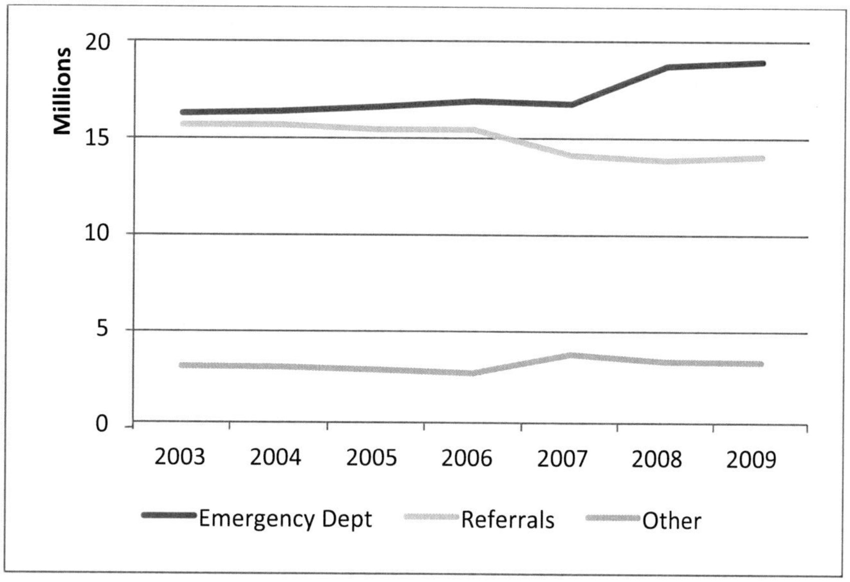

Source: National Hospital Discharge Survey
Note: Excludes live births. Weighted counts with imputed values.

As a result of these offsetting trends, by 2009, inpatient admissions from EDs accounted for roughly *half* of all inpatient admissions in the United States in 2009 (excluding live births) (see Figure 4.2). Not surprisingly, few elective admissions enter U.S. hospitals through EDs. However, two-thirds of non-elective inpatient admissions do.[8]

---

[8] An analysis of the NIS data showed that 66 percent of non-elective inpatient admissions are from the ED.

Figure 4.2. Share of Inpatient Admissions, by Source, 2009

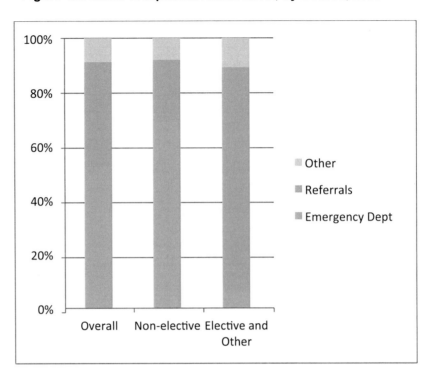

Source: National Hospital Discharge Survey
Note: Totals exclude live births. Weighted counts with imputed values.

2. Between 2003 and 2009, nearly all of the growth in hospital admissions was due to a 5.3 percent increase in non-elective admissions, which grew from 25.3 million in 2003 to 26.7 million in 2009.[9] Between 2003 and 2009, elective inpatient admissions and admissions from other sources remained flat. Note that these totals exclude live births (see Figure 4.3 and Appendix A, Table A.6, available online).

---

[9] The NIS data showed a similar change over time. Non-elective hospital admissions grew from 24.6 million in 2003 to 26.2 million in 2009.

Figure 4.3. Trends in Elective and Non-Elective Hospital Admissions, 2003–2009

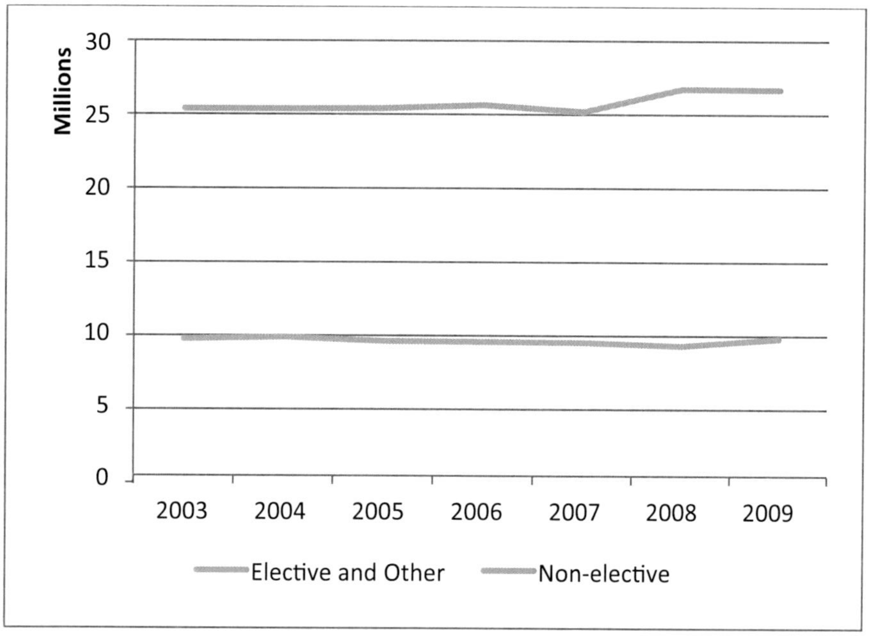

Source: National Hospital Discharge Survey
Note: Excludes live births. Weighted counts with imputed values.

What are the sources driving growth of non-elective inpatient admissions?

1. Between 2003 and 2009, nearly all of the growth in non-elective inpatient admissions was due to a marked increase in the number of inpatient admissions from hospital EDs. Over this seven-year interval, non-elective ED admissions grew by 20 percent, from 15.3 million in 2003 to 18.4 million in 2009.[10] This rate of growth was 3.8 times faster than growth of the U.S. population during the same time period. While non-elective admissions from EDs increased, non-elective admissions from private physician offices and clinics *declined* by 24 percent, from 8.0 million in 2003 to 6.1 million in 2009. Admissions from other sources, such as transfers from other facilities and law enforcement agencies, remained stable (see Figure 4.4 and Appendix A, Table A.6, available online).

---

[10] The NIS data showed that non-elective ED admissions grew from 15.9 million in 2003 to 17.3 million in 2009.

27

Figure 4.4. Trends in Non-Elective Hospital Admissions, by Source, 2003–2009

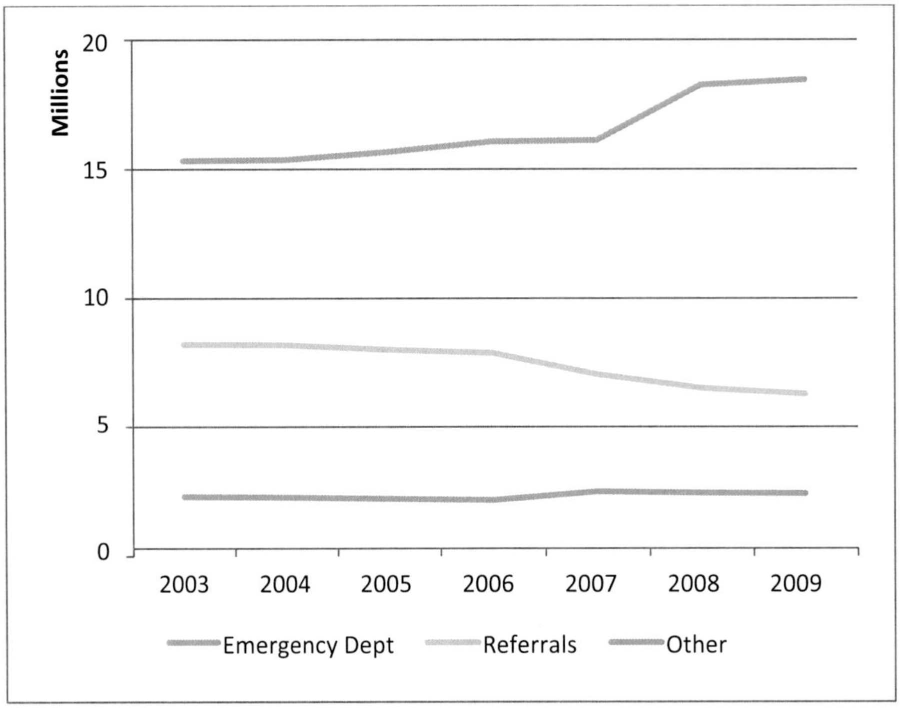

Source: National Hospital Discharge Survey
Note: Excludes live births. Weighted counts with imputed values.

2. Between 2003 and 2009, the fraction of non-elective inpatient admissions entering the hospital through the ED increased from 61 percent to 69 percent.[11] This represents an increase of 3.1 million ED admissions. Over the same time period, the proportion of non-elective admissions originating in doctors' offices and from outside referrals fell from 32 percent of non-elective admissions to 23 percent, a decrease of 1.9 million. Admissions from other sources, such as inter-facility transfers, remained stable (see Figure 4.5 and Appendix A, Table A.5, available online).

---

[11] The NIS data showed a lesser change. Between 2003 and 2009, the fraction of non-elective inpatient admissions entering the hospital through the ED increased from 65 percent in 2003 to 66 percent in 2009.

Figure 4.5. Share of Non-Elective Inpatient Admissions, 2003–2009

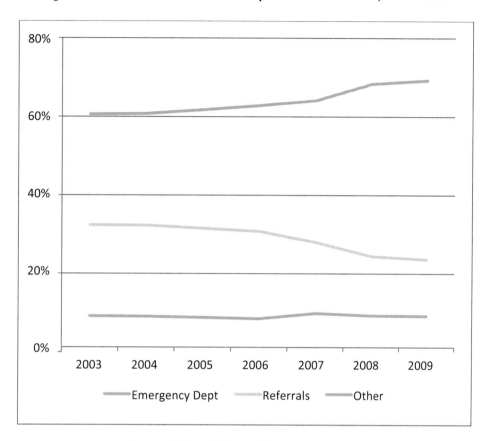

Source: National Hospital Discharge Survey
Note: Excludes live births. Weighted counts with imputed values. The standard errors for percentages are in Appendix A, Table A.10, available online. The standard errors for main results for Aims 1 and 2 and are very small— the standard errors are at most 0.25 percent, so the 95 percent confidence interval is ± 0.5 percent.

Why are primary care physicians admitting fewer patients to hospitals?

To gain insight into why PCPs appear to be sending more of their patients to EDs, rather than admitting non-elective cases directly from their offices, we analyzed the CTS Physician Survey (2004–05), and the 2008 HSC Health Tracking Physician Study. We supplemented these analyses with patient-level data collected by the 2003 CTS, the only edition of this survey to explore patient experiences with care-seeking in their communities.

1. One in 5 PCPs (20 percent) who responded to the 2004–05 CTS reported that they were unable to obtain non-emergency hospital admissions for *non-elective* admissions that they felt were medically necessary. In 2008, 22 percent of responding PCPs gave the same response.
2. Lack of qualified service providers or facilities was a relatively unimportant reason why they were unable to obtain non-emergency hospital admissions for some patients (see Figure 4.6). Only 37 percent of physician respondents to the CTS identified this factor as being "moderately" or "very" important.

In contrast, 75 percent of physicians indicated that health plan networks and

29

administrative barriers that limited patient access were "moderately important" or "very important" factors hindering their ability to obtain hospital admission for non-elective patients who did not require immediate stabilization in an ED. Seventy percent of physicians cited the patient's lack of health insurance or inadequate insurance coverage as a "moderately important" or "very important" factor in hindering their ability to secure non-emergency hospital admission.

Figure 4.6. Reasons Why Physicians Were Unable to Obtain Non-Emergency Hospital Admissions

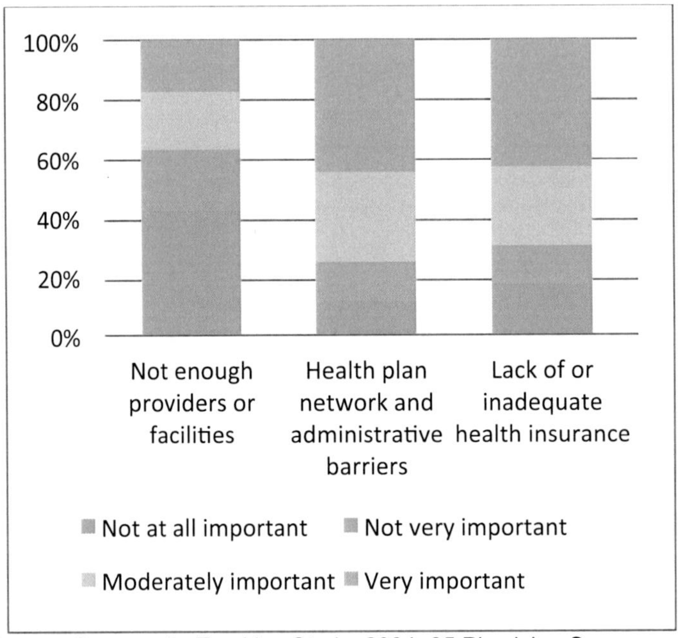

Source: Community Tracking Study, 2004–05 Physician Survey
Note: "Missing" responses are excluded from percent reported

In our interviews with PCPs, we asked whether they faced barriers to directly admitting non-elective patients to the hospital. Many said that they did, and noted that in such circumstances, the safest and easiest course of action is to send the patient to the ED. The most commonly cited reason discussants cited for referring patients to EDs rather than directly to hospitals involved clinical concerns, such as the severity or complexity of the patient's illness. The PCPs we interviewed also expressed concern that some patients could not tolerate the potentially lengthy wait for the direct admission process to unfold without ongoing medical attention. Many see a benefit to sending complex patients who need significant diagnostic testing to the ED, where technology and consultants are more readily available. Other reasons cited included the time required to arrange a direct admission and the need for clinical information that might not be available to a covering physician or practice partner after hours or on weekends.

Asked why more patients are being admitted through the ED than before, PCPs cited the growing shortage of primary care providers, group practices (where a providers may be on call but unfamiliar with their partner's patient), and the relative ease of sending a patient to the ED. Additionally, primary care providers cited patients' self-referral as a common reason why their patients end up in an ED for evaluation and admission, rather than coming to see them in the office.

Why are patients using EDs for non-urgent care?

1. Seventy-eight percent of respondents to the 2003 CTS survey reported making no ED visits in the prior 12 months. This statistic is roughly in line with self-reported ED use within the United States overall (CDC, 2012) (see Figure 4.7). Fourteen percent of survey respondents reported ED visit in the prior 12 months, 4.25 percent reported two visits, 1.76 percent reported three visits, 0.76 percent had four, and 1.25 percent reported that they had made five or more ED visits. The reported number of ED visits by year was stable over several years of the CTS survey. This suggests that the overall pattern of ED utilization by the U.S. population has not changed dramatically over time (Figure 4.7).

Figure 4.7. Number of Emergency Department Visits, by Year

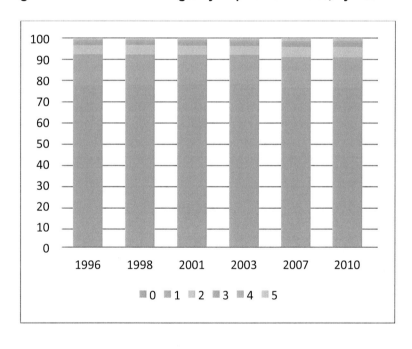

Source: Community Tracking Study, 1996, 1998, 2001, 2003, 2007, and 2010
Note: Number of ED Visits in Prior 12 Months by CTS Survey Participants

2. In 2003, the CTS asked respondents whose last ED visit was for a health problem *other* than an accident/injury whether they had been able to contact their doctor or another health professional before they sought care in an ED (see Figure 4.8). The majority who answered this question (58 percent) reported that they were unable to contact their doctor or another health professional. However, of these, only 15 percent made an actual attempt to contact their doctor before going to an ED. This implies that 49 percent of respondents who sought ED care did not attempt to contact a doctor or another health professional before heading to an ED. Of those who did not attempt contact, only 12 percent said that

31

they were aware of other places they could have gone for care. Interestingly, four out of five of those who contacted a health care professional were advised to go to an ED (Figure 4.8).

Figure 4.8. Efforts to Identify Non-Emergency Department Options for Acute Care, 2003

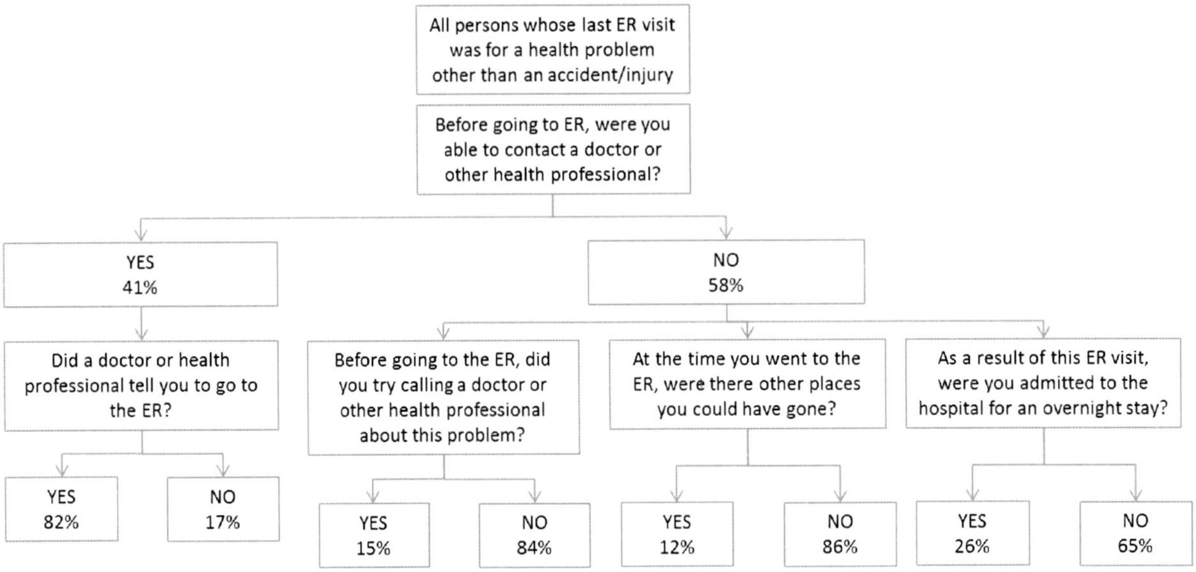

3. The 2010 edition of the CTS asked respondents whether they had a usual source of care, whether their health care providers offered office hours at night or on the weekends, and how difficult it was for them to contact a health care provider after regular office hours in the event that they need urgent medical care. Seventy percent of respondents reported that they had a usual source of care, while 28 percent did not (2 percent did not answer the question). Of those respondents who reported a usual source of care, 16 percent said that they had tried to contact their provider after regular office hours for an urgent medical need. Slightly more than half reported that their health care provider offers office hours at night or on weekends.

Thirty-two percent of patients who stated that their provider does not offer night or weekend hours reported that it was "very difficult" or "somewhat difficult" to contact a doctor or another health care provider with an after-hours concern. Conversely, only 11 percent of respondents whose provider offers office hours at night or on the weekends reported that they experienced a similar degree of difficulty contacting a doctor or other health care provider after hours (see Figure 4.9).

Figure 4.9. Usual Source of Care and Difficulty to Contact Provider After-Hours

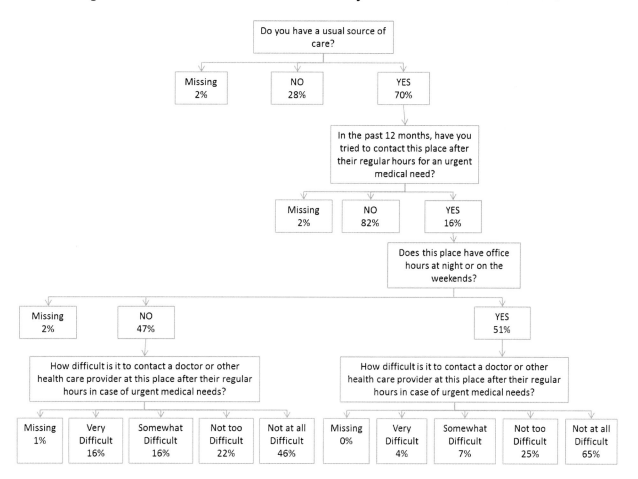

Does a patient's insurance coverage influence likelihood of admission and his/her portal of entry to inpatient care?

1. Medicare accounts for the largest single share of inpatient admissions, counting both elective and non-elective admissions. However, the most important source of inpatient admissions varies by the patient's primary insurance. For example, a majority of privately insured patients (elective and non-elective cases) are directly admitted from their doctors' office or a clinic. However, 60 percent of all inpatient admissions of Medicare beneficiaries and nearly half (47 percent) of inpatient admissions of Medicaid beneficiaries enter the hospital through the ED. Less than a quarter of uninsured patients are admitted from a doctor's office, clinic or other sources. Nearly three out of every four uninsured patients (73 percent) are admitted from an ED (see Figure 4.10).

Figure 4.10. All Inpatient Admissions, by Primary Payer and Source, 2009

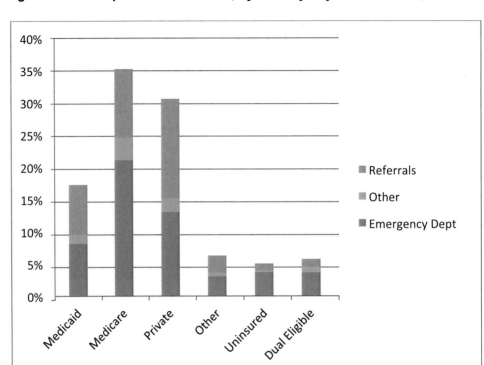

Source: National Hospital Discharge Survey
Note: Excludes live births. Weighted counts with imputed values.

2. Between 2003 and 2009, the proportion of inpatients admitted through the ED increased across all major payer groups. Although the fraction of inpatient admissions varies by primary payer, all payer groups showed upward trends in the annual proportion of patients admitted through the ED (see Figure 4.11).

Figure 4.11. Share of All Inpatients Admitted Through the Emergency Department, by Primary Payer, 1993–2009

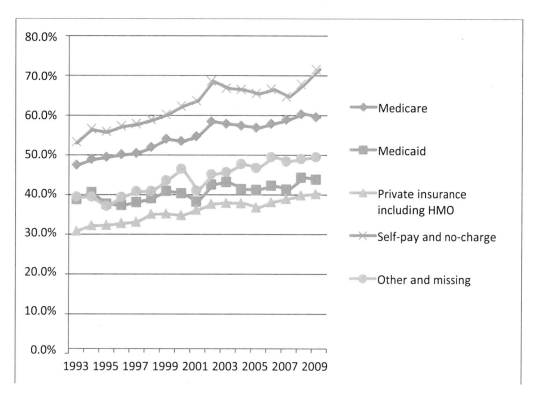

Data Source: Nationwide Inpatient Sample
Note: Excludes live births. Weighted counts.

3. Over the past 16 years, Medicare has consistently been the top primary payer for hospitals, accounting for 38 percent to 41 percent of all inpatients. Private insurance is the second-most common primary payer, although it has declined from a high of 37 percent of inpatients in 1999 to a low of 32 percent in 2009. The downward trend in employer-sponsored insurance as a primary payer is likely due to the progressive erosion of such insurance throughout the decade, followed by dramatic job losses in 2009. The share of inpatients admitted to the hospital with Medicaid as their primary payer varied from a low of 15 percent in 1997 to a high of 18 percent in 2009, when Medicaid enrollments nationwide jumped as stimulus funds were used to buffer the dramatic loss of employer-sponsored insurance. As a result of these offsetting effects, the proportion of hospital admissions involving self-pay and no-charge patients stayed relatively constant, at 5–6 percent of inpatient admissions (Figure 4.12).

Figure 4.12. Primary Payer for All Hospital Admissions, 1993–2009

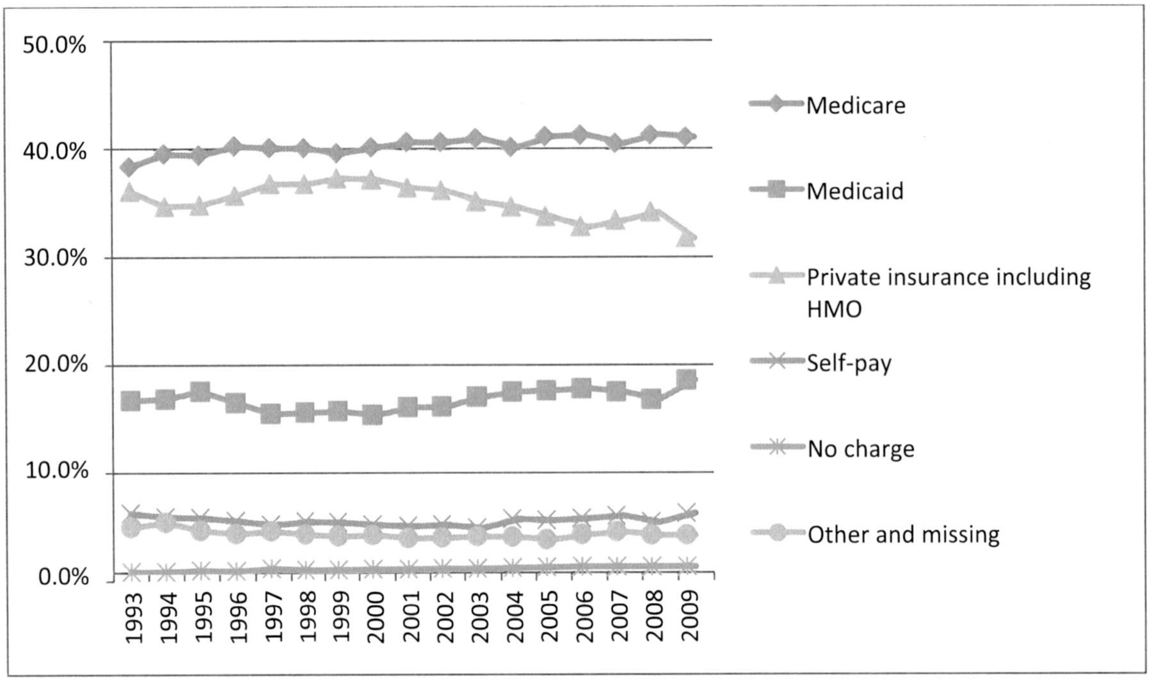

Source: Nationwide Inpatient Sample, 1993–2009

4. From 1993 and 2009, Medicare was the dominant primary payer for ED admissions. Over this time period, the proportion of ED admissions involving Medicare beneficiaries grew modestly (Figure 4.13), while the fraction of ED admissions covered by private insurance decreased slightly, dipping more in 2009 with the onset of the recession. The proportion of ED admissions covered by Medicaid admissions was generally stable—with the exception of 2009, when stimulus funds were used to boost enrollment in Medicaid to blunt what would have been an even greater increase in self-pay admissions due to the millions of workers who lost their jobs and health insurance.

**Figure 4.13. Primary Payer for Inpatient Admissions
Originating in Emergency Departments, 1993–2009**

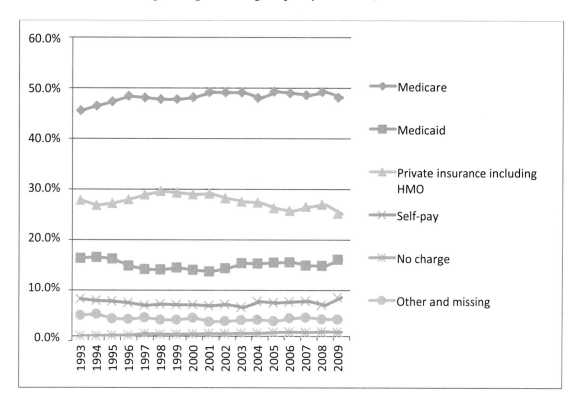

Source: Nationwide Inpatient Sample (NIS), 1993–2009

5. The modest growth in Medicare admissions through EDs appears to be a product of rising numbers of beneficiaries, rather than higher rates of admission. This suggests that growth in Medicare admissions is a product of the aging baby boom generation, not more aggressive hospitalization of Medicare beneficiaries. Between 1999 and 2009, population rates of hospitalization by major payer per 100 beneficiary-years were relatively constant (Figure 4.14).

**Figure 4.14. Population Rates of Inpatient Admissions
from Emergency Departments, 1999–2009**

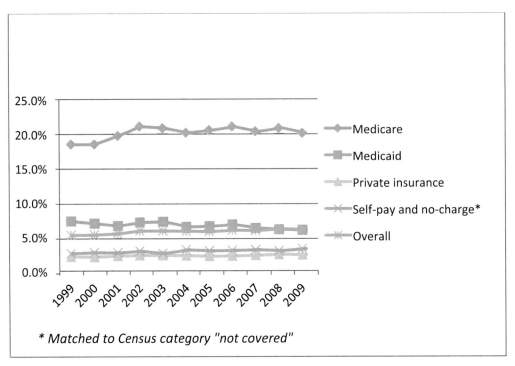

* Matched to Census category "not covered"

Source: Nationwide Inpatient Sample (NIS), 1999–2009.Denominators are population counts of individuals by primary insurance coverage (private, Medicaid, Medicare, self pay/no charge) by year. Data from the Current Population Survey Annual Social and Economic Supplements (CPS ASEC, Census 2011).

6. In contrast to the slight growth in Medicare admissions from EDs, population rates of Medicare and Medicaid admissions from non-ED sources (predominantly, physician offices) declined steeply (Figure 4.15). The declines among privately insured patients and the small percentage of uninsured patients admitted from non-ED sources were more modest. As noted earlier in our results, and reinforced by the comments we heard in our focus groups and individual interviews with PCPs, this decrease appears to be driven by a change in how patients are being admitted to the hospital, rather than a sharply reduced need to admit patients. Our interview participants advised us that for a variety of reasons, they are more likely to send acutely ill patients to the ED for stabilization and admission workup than they were in the past.

**Figure 4.15. Population Rates of Inpatient Admission
from Non–Emergency Department Sources, 1999–2009**

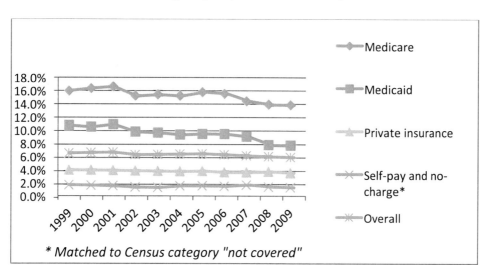

Matched to Census category "not covered"

Source: Nationwide Inpatient Sample (NIS), 1999-2009. Denominators are population counts by primary insurance coverage (private, Medicaid, Medicare, self pay/no charge) by year from the Current Population Survey Annual Social and Economic Supplements (CPS ASEC, Census 2011).

Does a patient's source of primary health insurance influence his/her probability of hospitalization from the ED?

1. The likelihood that an ED patient will be hospitalized varies substantially by primary payer. Not surprisingly, given their age and the higher prevalence of comorbid conditions, Medicare beneficiaries (which account for 20 percent of all ED visits), are 3.4 times more likely to be hospitalized at the end of ED visits than privately insured patients, who are typically younger and tend to have better baseline health. Although it appears at first glance that Medicaid patients are less likely to be admitted than privately insured patients, this difference disappeared after our analysis was adjusted for patient gender and age. Uninsured patients were much less likely to be hospitalized, even after standardizing the analysis for group differences in age and gender (Table 4.1).

Some may speculate that this difference may be explained if uninsured patients are more often admitted to a different acute care hospital (as sometimes occurs when a self-pay ED patient is transferred from a private hospital to a public hospital). However, this does not appear to be the case. In 2009, about 167,000 self-pay patients were admitted to a second hospital, representing about 11 percent of acute care hospital admissions of self-pay patients. However, a similar percentage of privately insured patients (12 percent) were admitted to a different acute care hospital as well, so accounting for these admissions would not narrow the difference in admission rates (source: 2009 NEDS, data not shown).

Table 4.1. Emergency Department Admissions, by Payer, 2009

Primary Payer	Disposition from ED		Total ED Visits	% of ED Visits	% of ED Admissions	Admission Rate (unadjusted)	Crude Rate Ratio**	Adjusted Rate Ratio**
	Not Admitted	Admitted*						
Medicare	16,203,253	9,736,591	25,939,845	20.1%	49.7%	37.5%	3.42	2.65
Medicaid	28,782,535	3,091,233	31,873,768	24.7%	15.8%	9.7%	0.88	1.11
Private insurance	37,784,362	4,650,736	42,435,098	32.9%	23.7%	11.0%	1.00	1.00
Self-pay	19,588,042	1,319,720	20,907,762	16.2%	6.7%	6.3%	0.58	0.50
No charge	994,629	165,408	1,160,037	0.9%	0.8%	14.3%	1.30	1.09
Other	5,452,254	605,458	6,057,712	4.7%	3.1%	10.0%	0.91	0.81
Missing or invalid	487,420	23,399	510,819	0.4%	0.1%	4.6%	0.42	0.36
Overall	109,292,495	19,592,545	128,885,040	100.0%	100.0%	15.2%		

Source: NEDS, weighted counts.
* Inpatient disposition is to same hospital.
** Private insurance referent; adjustment using direct standardization.

Does a patient's type of insurance influence a primary care physician's decision to send the patient to the ED?

We also asked our focus group and interview participants specifically about the role of insurance in influencing whether the physician sent the patient to the ED versus directly admitting the patient. Nearly all of the physicians we interviewed insisted that the type of insurance a patient has does not influence their decision. Only one physician identified insurance as an issue hindering his ability to achieve a direct admission.

Do plans that offer care coordination have lower rates of inpatient admission from EDs than fee-for-service plans?

As described in our methods section, AHRQ staff ran a preliminary analysis of their SEDD file that was restricted to 20 states that code patients covered by a Medicare Advantage Plan differently than those covered by Medicare FFS (Mutter R., personal communication). Not surprisingly, the logistic regression revealed that the odds of hospital admission increased significantly with the age of the patient. Female Medicare beneficiaries were less likely to be hospitalized than men. Hospital status also mattered, with inpatient admission more likely if the patient was seen in the EDs of an urban hospital, a teaching hospital, or a for-profit hospital, even after adjusting for other comorbidities. However, once all of these factors were controlled for, the likelihood of ED admission was not associated with coverage by Medicare Choice relative to traditional Medicare FFS (adjusted Odds Ratio: 0.993, 95% CI: 0.905–1.090).

AHRQ staff repeated the analysis with a dataset limited to CCS categories and found that, in certain circumstances, clinicians might consider "judgment calls" regarding whether to admit the patient. These CCS categories include: 122 (pneumonia), 108 (congestive heart failure), 127 (COPD), 102 (nonspecific chest pain), 237 (complications of a device, graft, or implant), 197 (skin and subcutaneous infection), 159 (urinary tract infection), and 55 (fluid and electrolyte disorders). After taking other potentially confounding variables into consideration, analysis of this subset revealed a trend towards lower odds of admission among Medicare Choice patients, but the 95 percent confidence interval did not exclude one (adjusted odds ratio: 0.921, 95% CI: 0.834–1.017).

Finally, AHRQ staff repeated the analysis a third time, calculating the adjusted odds of admission from the ED for each of the CCS conditions in turn. This analysis found slightly lower adjusted odds of admission among Medicare Choice patients diagnosed with pneumonia, or fluid and electrolyte disorders; no change in adjusted odds of admission patients with congestive heart failure, urinary tract infections, or complications of a device, graft, or implant; and slightly higher adjusted odds of admission for patients with COPD, nonspecific chest pain, skin and subcutaneous infections (data not shown). Viewed collectively, these analyses offer little support for the hypotheses that patients covered by plans with a greater level of care coordination are less likely to be hospitalized relative to those covered by a traditional FFS plan, at least among the Medicare population. Unfortunately, AHRQ's team does not feel that the state-level coding is sufficiently robust (yet) to allow for a valid comparison of admission rates of ED patients covered by a private HMO or Managed care plan, or Medicaid Managed Care (Mutter R, Personal Communication).

Comments from our focus group participants provide additional context to these observations. Participants in both the ED and hospitalist focus groups reported that although clinical considerations have the greatest weight in their admission decisions, non-clinical issues, such as the patients' safety at home, the availability of family or social-services support, and timely access to follow-up care are also important. Several participants noted that when care coordination is available, such as when an ED case manager is on duty, they feel more confident that adequate follow-up arrangements can be made, so they may be more willing to discharge a fragile or borderline patient.

Are EDs playing a role in reducing preventable hospital admissions?

For a number of years, AHRQ has monitored hospitalization rates for patients with "ambulatory care sensitive conditions," such as asthma, congestive heart failure, diabetes, and pediatric gastroenteritis (Kruzikas, 2000), as an indicator of the accessibility and quality of primary care in the United States. To formalize this process, AHRQ identified a standard set of admission diagnoses as "prevention quality indicators" (PQI) (Davies et al., 2009). Between 2000 and 2006, such "potentially preventable" hospitalizations for chronic conditions decreased by 11 percent in the United States, from 1,213 to 1,078 hospitalizations per 100,000 adults) (U.S. DHHS, 2009). At the time the AHRQ report was released, this observation was interpreted as evidence that primary care is doing a more effective job of managing patients with ACS conditions. However, it is also possible that this reduction is due to the more active management of patients with these conditions in the ED (to treat and discharge rather than admit to the hospital).

As health care financing shifts from FFS to such funding mechanisms as bundled payments, Accountable Care Organizations, and various forms of risk-sharing or capitation, financial incentives for health care systems and health plans may be more fully aligned to reduce hospital admissions, rather than to promote them as an important source of health system revenue. To look for early signals that this is happening, we undertook a preliminary analysis to determine whether or not aggressive treatment by ED staff, followed by discharge, might be moderating growth of hospital admissions of patients with ACS conditions, such as asthma, diabetes, and heart failure.

We analyzed rates of admission for ACS conditions from 2000 to 2009.

Table 4.2. AHRQ Prevention Quality Indicators Conditions and Composites

Overall Composite (PQI #90)

- PQI #01 Diabetes Short-Term Complications
- PQI #03 Diabetes Long-Term Complications
- PQI #05 COPD or Asthma in Older Adults
- PQI #07 Hypertension
- PQI #08 Heart Failure
- PQI #10 Dehydration

- PQI #11 Bacterial Pneumonia
- PQI #12 Urinary Tract Infection
- PQI #13 Angina without Procedure
- PQI #14 Uncontrolled Diabetes
- PQI #15 Asthma in Younger Adults
- PQI #16 Lower-Extremity Amputation Among Patients With Diabetes

Acute Composite (PQI #91)

- PQI #10 Dehydration
- PQI #11 Bacterial Pneumonia

- PQI #12 Urinary Tract Infection

Chronic Composite (PQI #92)

- PQI #01 Diabetes Short-Term Complications
- PQI #03 Diabetes Long-Term Complications
- PQI #05 COPD or Asthma in Older Adults
- PQI #07 Hypertension
- PQI #08 Congestive Heart Failure

- PQI #13 Angina without Procedure
- PQI #14 Uncontrolled Diabetes
- PQI #15 Asthma in Younger Adults
- PQI #16 Lower-Extremity Amputation Among Patients With Diabetes

Source: (AHRQ, 2012).

During this period, the ED's total share of PQI-related inpatient admissions increased from 70 percent to 79 percent. This shift was also reflected in changing numbers of PQI admissions from non-ED to ED sources, depicted in Table 4.3.

**Table 4.3. Trends in PQI-related Inpatient Admissions,
by Source, 2000, 2005, and 2009**

	2000	2005	2009	% Change 2000–2009
Total non-elective admissions – all sources	23,051,221	25,484,263	26,207,448	**14%**
Total Composite PQI admissions- all sources	4,028,234	4,157,656	4,038,293	**0%**
Total non-elective admissions - ED	13,623,038	15,867,649	17,257,291	**27%**
Acute PQIs	1,094,902	328,306	1,258,593	15%
Chronic PQIs	1,727,538	1,757,100	1,930,608	12%
Overall Composite PQIs	2,822,584	3,085,397	3,189,444	**13%**
Total non-elective admissions - non-ED	9,428,184	9,616,614	8,950,158	-5%
Acute PQIs	441,372	442,769	326,936	-26%
Chronic PQIs	764,582	629,615	522,203	-32%
Overall Composite PQI	1,205,650	1,072,259	848,849	-30%

Source: NIS, weighted counts.

Note: According to the AHRQ, "The Prevention Quality Indicators (PQI) are measures of potentially avoidable hospitalizations for ACS Conditions (ACSCs), which, though they rely on hospital discharge data, are intended to reflect issues of access to, and quality of, ambulatory care in a given geographic area. The PQI composites are intended to improve the statistical precision of the individual PQI, allowing for greater discrimination in performance among areas and improved ability to identify potentially determining factors in performance. An overall composite captures the general concept of potentially avoidable hospitalization connecting the individual PQI measures, which are all rates at the area level. Separate composite measures were created for acute and chronic conditions to investigate different factors influencing hospitalization rates for each condition." (AHRQ, 2012).

The composite measure for acute PQIs includes dehydration; bacterial pneumonia; and urinary tract infections. The composite measure for chronic PQIs includes diabetes (short-term and long-term complications), COPD or asthma in older adults; hypertension; congestive heart failure, angina; uncontrolled diabetes; asthma in younger adults; and lower-extremity amputation among patients with diabetes. (AHRQ, 2012).

Between 2000 and 2009, non-elective admissions to U.S. hospitals grew by 14 percent overall, while PQI-related admissions remained flat. This was due, in part, to a dramatic decline in PQI admissions from non-ED sources (a 30 percent drop between 2000 and 2009) and a slower-than-expected rise in PQI admissions from EDs, given overall growth of ED visits and non-elective ED admissions. During the time that non-elective admissions from the ED grew by 27 percent, PQI-related admissions increased at half that rate (13 percent).

There are two possible explanations for the sharp decline in non-ED admissions with ACS conditions (PQIs). One is that primary care providers did a better job of managing patients with ACS conditions, thereby reducing flares of their illness and the subsequent need for inpatient admission. The other, equally plausible explanation is that the reduction of PQI-related admissions from doctors' offices and other non-ED settings was largely due to the growing tendency of office-based practitioners to send acutely ill patients to an ED rather than directly admitting the patient to the hospital. The comments made during our interviews with ED, hospitalist, and primary care physicians support the latter explanation.

Either way, the news is encouraging. Lack of growth of inpatient admissions related to PQIs between 2000 and 2009 stands in stark contrast to the overall growth of non-elective admissions (14 percent), and the even sharper increase in non-elective admissions from the ED (27 percent). These data suggest that EDs might have played a more positive role in constraining growth of potentially preventable hospital admissions than was previously realized (Russo, Jiang, & Barrett, 2007).

To gain further insight into these trends, we examined rates of ED visits and hospital admissions for ACS conditions using the CCS system. This is a disease categorization scheme that collapses the ICD-9-CM diagnosis codes into 260 mutually exclusive, clinically meaningful categories. We used the coding that was available in the NEDS to determine the percent of ED visits by primary and secondary CCS categories that were admitted to the same hospital for years 2006 to 2009.

Table 4.4. PQIs Paired with Corresponding CCS Conditions

Conditions	Sources
PQI – Diabetes short term complication + Uncontrolled diabetes	All inpatient admissions
CCS – Diabetes mellitus with complications	ED visits + inpatient admits from ED
PQI – COPD or asthma in older adults + asthma in younger adults	All inpatient admissions
CCS –COPD and bronchiectasis + asthma	ED visits + inpatient admits from ED
PQI – Urinary tract infection	All inpatient admissions
CCS – Diseases of the urinary system	ED visits + inpatient admits from ED
PQI – Hypertension	All inpatient admissions
CCS – Hypertension	ED visits + inpatient admits from ED
PQI – Congestive heart failure + angina	All inpatient admissions
CCS – Diseases of the heart	ED visits + inpatient admits from ED
PQI – Dehydration	All inpatient admissions
CCS – Fluid and electrolyte disorders	ED visits + inpatient admits from ED

Looking at all primary CCS categories, we determined that between 15.2 percent and 15.5 percent of ED visits resulted in admission to the same hospital, a figure in line with the national rate of ED admissions rate reported by the National Hospital Ambulatory Medical Survey–ED subsample (NHAMCS-ED). The CCS categories associated with the highest percentage of ED visits resulting in inpatient admissions (to the same hospital) are diseases of the circulatory system (40–44 percent) and endocrine, nutritional, and metabolic diseases and immunity

45

disorders (38–39 percent). The CCS categories with the lowest percentage of ED visits resulting in inpatient admission include diseases of the nervous system and sense organs (about 6 percent) and other (about 9 percent). There was minimal variation over time for the CCS categories presented.

To determine what might have accounted for growth of ED admissions involving patients with ACS conditions (i.e., PQIs), we selected secondary CCS categories that correspond reasonably well with their associated AHRQ-designated PQIs (see Table 4.4). This allowed us to approximate whether rising numbers of ED admissions due to various PQIs of interest were the result of higher numbers of ED visits, a lower threshold for admitting patients with those conditions, or a greater number of referrals of ill patients from doctor's offices.

As Table 4.5 suggests, it appears that for most of the comparisons we made, ED visits did not increase to the same degree as ED admissions for the related CCS. The notable exceptions to this trend were admissions related to heart failure and angina, which declined despite an increase in ED visits for these conditions. ED admissions for hypertension decreased as well. We suspect, but cannot definitively prove, that this is due to the impact of ED observation units and perhaps the growing tendency of some ED providers and hospital physicians to admit borderline cases to "observation status" on an inpatient ward. Because neither disposition is currently coded in NIS or NEDS datasets, we cannot address this possibility.

Table 4.5. CCS Percent Change from 2006 to 2009

	2006	2009	% Change 2006–2009
CCS – Diabetes mellitus with complications			
Number of ED Visits	710,846	764,068	+7.5%
Number of Hospital Admissions	361,884	407,490	+12.6%
ED Admission Rate	50.9%	53.3%	↑4.7%
CCS – COPD and bronchiectasis + asthma			
Number of ED Visits	3,459,911	3,941,599	+13.9%
Number of Hospital Admissions	765,440	933,509	+22.0%
ED Admission Rate	22.1%	23.7%	↑7.2%
CCS – Diseases of the urinary system			
Number of ED Visits	4,841,847	5,314,274	+9.8%
Number of Hospital Admissions	891,167	982,458	+10.2%
ED Admission Rate	18.4%	18.5%	↑0.5%
CCS – Hypertension			
Number of ED Visits	779,671	934,280	+19.8%
Number of Hospital Admissions	224,628	249,102	+10.9%
ED Admission Rate	28.8%	26.7%	↓6.3%
CCS – Diseases of the heart			
Number of ED Visits	7,583,340	7,954,331	+4.9%
Number of Hospital Admissions	3,168,737	2,987,344	-5.7%
ED Admission Rate	41.8%	37.6%	↓10%
CCS – Fluid and electrolyte disorders			
Number of ED Visits	909,276	925,045	+1.7%
Number of Hospital Admissions	355,027	379,641	+6.9%
ED Admission Rate	39.0%	41.0%	↑5%

Source: NEDS for CCS.
Note: Weighted counts. Share continuing to inpatient is for same hospital.

In our view, the overall growth of ED visits involving ACS CCS conditions, at a time when admissions from doctors' offices were falling, and the relatively modest increase in admission rates associated with these CCS codes compared to the past, suggest that office-based physicians are sending probable admissions to the ED with increasing frequency rather than directly admitting them from their office, as in the past. Comments offered by members of our three focus groups and by individual PCPs we interviewed support this view. The strongest evidence that ED care may be exerting a moderating effect on potentially preventable admissions may be seen in the declining number and rate of hospital admissions due to heart failure and angina (see

Table 4.5). This is likely due to the introduction and diffusion of ED observation units (Schuur & Venkatesh, 2012).

Qualitative data from our focus groups and interviews support these findings. Although participants readily conceded that aggressive ED workups and treatment are costly (and might be needed less often if ED physicians and hospitalists could routinely gain access to their patients' electronic medical record) interviewees asserted that EDs help hold down growth of health care costs by providing stabilizing care and preventing some inpatient admissions.

5. Discussion

Assessing the Value of Emergency Department Care

The high costs and less-than-ideal outcomes produced by America's health care system have led policymakers and payers to examine the value of various tests, treatments, and procedures (Morgan et al., 2012). In this context, value is generally defined as "health outcomes achieved per dollar spent" (Morgan et al., 2012; Porter, 2010; Porter & Teisberg, 2006).

Measurement of value in health care is relatively new and depends, in large part, on whether it is determined from the viewpoint of patients, insurers, or society. Patients want, most of all, to have a good treatment outcome and to be free from harm. Those who are insured care much less about the price. Payers want the lowest price for an acceptable outcome. Society wants health care providers to improve the health of its members at an aggregate cost that doesn't crowd out other important priorities.

EDs play a pivotal role in the delivery of acute ambulatory and inpatient care. That role has evolved in response to economic, clinical, and political pressures. Because EDs charge higher prices for minor illness and injury care than other ambulatory care settings, ED care is frequently characterized as "the most expensive care there is." But this depiction ignores the many roles that EDs play, and the statutory obligation of hospital EDs to provide care to all in need without regard for their ability to pay.

Our study confirms, as the IOM Emergency Care Committee and other groups have noted, that hospital EDs serve a wide range of societal roles. These include, first and foremost, provision of life-saving care to critically ill and injured patients. But increasingly, EDs are also being used to facilitate the assessment and management of patients who need non-elective admission, to perform complex evaluations of high-risk patients, to provide acute care to insured and uninsured Americans who cannot get timely access to care elsewhere, and (for approximately 60 million low-income or uninsured Americans and many undocumented immigrants) to fulfill their congressionally mandated obligation to serve as "the safety net of the safety net." To meet these different and sometimes conflicting roles, emergency physicians and nurses must be prepared to manage a wide range of problems and concerns.

Because the core mission of EDs is stabilization of patients with potentially life-threatening illnesses and injuries, they must always be prepared, on a moment's notice, to provide lifesaving emergency care to an afflicted individual or a community that has sustained a sudden mass-casualty event. But the bulk of ED activity is devoted to managing unscheduled, high-acuity visits by patients with acute undifferentiated complaints. Our analysis also confirms that EDs have become the primary entry portal for inpatient admissions, the main source of revenue for most hospitals. In some safety net hospitals and trauma centers, ED admissions may account for

60–70 percent of the facility's inpatient volume (Delia & Cantor, 2009). More frequently, office-based physicians are beginning to direct their patients to the ED, rather than directly admitting the patient themselves.

EDs are responsible for essentially all the recent growth of hospital admissions, and now account for approximately half of hospital inpatients in the United States, excluding live births. Since inpatient care accounts for more than 30 percent of aggregate U.S. health care spending—nearly a trillion dollars per year—this means that decisions made in EDs have a profound impact on the financial fortunes of hospitals on one hand, and the aggregate costs of health care on the other.

In terms of fiscal consequences, the role of EDs in facilitating or preventing hospital admissions is most consequential. Numerically, however, ED staff members devote more time and aggregate resources to the provision of outpatient care. In any given year, one out of five Americans makes at least one visit to an ED (CDC, 2012; Owens et al., 2010). Because EDs are often a community's only source of treatment that is readily available after hours and on weekends, they manage 11 percent of all outpatient visits in the United States and fully 28 percent of all acute care visits, focusing disproportionately on those involving more dangerous or worrisome symptoms, such as chest pain, abdominal pain, dyspnea, and severe headache (Pitts et al., 2010).

EDs are organized to provide ready access without an appointment, and typically manage patients otherwise followed by other physicians. Thus, it is extremely difficult to isolate the effects of ED treatment from the interventions that took place before, or occur after, an ED encounter. When a patient with vague chest pain is found to have signs of acute cardiac ischemia and is rushed to the catheterization lab for emergency angioplasty, should their good outcome be attributable to timely diagnosis by the ED physician, or the cardiologist's subsequent procedure? When a patient with abdominal pain is carefully evaluated and found not to require exploratory surgery, are the savings (and potential complications that were avoided) attributable to the ED, or was the extensive workup unreasonable? If a patient with asthma is treated in an ED-based observation unit for 12 hours, and successfully discharged home, is the avoided admission "credited" to the ED, or the ongoing efforts (including prompt follow up) of the patient's PCP? These challenges, and the limited funds dedicated to date to health services research in EDs, explain why little progress has been made in quantifying the value of ED care (Institute of Medicine, 2006; Morgan et al., 2012).

The Evolving Relationship Between EDs and Primary Care Providers

Our findings indicate that the relationship between hospital EDs and PCPs is changing rapidly. This is likely due, in part, to the growing shortage of PCPs as well as the growing differentiation of generalist practice into two groups: PCPs who largely restrict their practice to their outpatient settings, and a second set of "hospitalist" physicians who focus on treating hospital inpatients. With hospitalists focusing on high-acuity inpatient care and emergency physicians specializing in high acuity and undifferentiated outpatient care, office-based physicians have less need and perhaps less desire to accommodate unscheduled visits by acutely ill patients.

There are practical considerations as well. In the modern era, it is not unusual for an office-based PCP to be scheduled to see 25–30 patients a day in 15-minute increments. If an acutely ill patient arrives unexpectedly, it can wreck the doctor's schedule (Stubbs, 2009). The time pressure on PCPs has grown so great, many regard any unscheduled visit, even one involving a relatively minor problem, as a disruption to their workday (Berenson & Rich, 2010). In such situations, it is much easier and arguably more prudent to direct the patient to a nearby ED (Institute of Medicine, 2006). Likewise, the inability to assure timely access to outpatient follow-up appears to be a factor in leading some emergency physicians to err on the side of caution and admit a borderline patient (Asplin et al., 2005). Our focus groups with emergency physicians, and our individual interviews with PCPs, support these observations.

Emergency Departments as Diagnostic Centers

Qualitative findings from our study also indicate that EDs are being increasingly used by PCPs to perform accelerated diagnostic workups of patients with potentially serious problems (Institute of Medicine, 2007). In a recently published paper, Pitts noted that in the past decade, "[An] increasingly strained primary care infrastructure for adults has resulted in greater use of the ED for first-contact care" (Pitts, 2012) Obvious advantages of this strategy include the fact that EDs have access to advanced diagnostic technology, including CT scanners, magnetic resonance imaging, and nuclear scans, rarely available in doctors' offices. ED staff also has more ready access to subspecialist consultants and interventionalists if needed. The downside of this strategy is that if the patient does not regularly receive care at that hospital or health care system, the emergency physician may be unable to access the patient's electronic medical record (A. L. Kellermann & Jones, 2013; Potini, Weerasuriya, Lowery-North, & Kellermann, 2011). Because ED physicians are expected to achieve a high level of diagnostic certainty, many compensate by repeating extensive blood work and ordering costly diagnostic tests (Pitts et al., 2012).

Their prudence may be justified. The three most common symptoms of Medicare patients who are ultimately *discharged* from EDs—abdominal pain, chest pain, and shortness of breath —can represent benign conditions or life-threatening disorders, such as acute myocardial infarction, bowel perforation, or a pulmonary embolus. Even a seemingly minor complaint in a younger, healthier individual can turn out to reflect a dangerous condition (Raven et al., 2013).

Do Emergency Departments Prevent Costly Inpatient Admissions?

Although payers and patients frequently complain about the high charges associated with ED visits, little thought is given to the costs avoided when an ED evaluation, or an intense period of treatment, avoids the need for a far more costly inpatient stay. The examples in the prior paragraph of potentially dangerous presenting symptoms are illustrative. Prior to the development of ED-based observation units, older patients with chest pain were routinely admitted to the hospital to "rule out" an acute myocardial infarction, a process that typically unfolded over a two- or even three-day hospital stay. Today, the same individuals can be comprehensively evaluated in an observation unit, with risk stratification, within 6–24 hours without ever seeing an inpatient bed (Amsterdam et al., 2010; Apple et al., 2005; Jaffe, Babuin, & Apple, 2006).

An early signal of the impact of this strategy was identified by Schuur and Ventakesh in their 2012 study that documented substantial growth in non-elective admissions from EDs. Of the 13 most common conditions for which patients are admitted from EDs to the hospital, they noted that one—coronary atherosclerosis—was associated with a declining number of admissions. They speculated that this was due to the recent adoption of rapid "rule-out" protocols and ED-based observation units (Schuur & Venkatesh, 2012).

As pressure builds to constrain further growth of health care spending, EDs are likely to come under greater scrutiny. Whereas policymakers and third party payers have largely focused on the cost of ED care relative to treatment in other outpatient settings, the role of EDs in either facilitating or preventing hospital admissions may be a bigger story. The average cost of an ED visit is $922 (Stranges, 2011). The average cost of an inpatient stay is ten times as much ($9,200 (Machlin, 2011; Stranges, 2011).

When health system and provider reimbursement shifts from FFS to bundled payments, capitation, and accountable care organizations, hospitals will be incentivized to avoid preventable inpatient admissions rather than encourage them. At that point, hospital administrators will shift from encouraging their ED staff to admit "borderline" patients to urging their ED staff to keep them out (Wiler et al., 2012). In the case of early readmissions of Medicare beneficiaries, this shift in emphasis has already occurred (Center for Medicare and Medicaid Services, 2013).

When and how ED care prevents hospitalizations has not been previously studied in detail. The notable exception, described earlier in this subsection, is chest pain (Amsterdam et al., 2010; Apple et al., 2005; Jaffe et al., 2006). Based on positive results with chest pain, directors of observation units are developing and implementing pathways for a wider array of conditions, including transient ischemic attack (near-stroke), asthma, and acute complications of diabetes (Baugh, Venkatesh, & Bohan, 2011; Venkatesh et al., 2011).

According to a 2006 AHRQ study, potentially preventable hospital admissions cost our nation more than $30 billion annually (Jiang, Russo, & Barrett, 2006). This suggests that in the future, EDs may be seen less as an important source of inpatient admissions, and more as the "final line of defense" to prevent costly inpatient admissions and readmissions. Our findings offer early evidence, albeit inconclusive, that EDs are already having a positive impact by constraining the growth of admissions involving AHRQ-identified PQIs.

Study Limitations

Within the limitations of the available data, we sought to characterize the evolving role of hospital EDs in our health care system. To achieve our specific aims, we analyzed large amounts of information from four national datasets maintained by the U.S. Department of Health and Human Services, and a series of privately funded, community-based surveys conducted by the Center for Studying Health System Change. To provide context for our observations, we also conducted focus groups and individual interviews with practicing emergency physicians, hospitalists, and emergency physicians. This multi-pronged approach provided a number of advantages; however, it was also limited in important respects.

Studies of secular trends, such as our analyses of varying numbers and rates of hospital admissions over time, are inevitably hampered by inadequacies in the data, and the inability of investigators to control for the numerous factors that can influence clinical practice and physician thinking over time. Although we are confident that our numbers reflect the aggregate impact of these influences on counts and population rates of hospital admission, we are less confident that we, or anyone, can precisely characterize the reasons behind them. This is equally true of our analysis of patients' care-seeking behavior. That issue is even less well studied than decisionmaking by physicians, and the data we analyzed from the Community Tracking Study are ten years old.

Although 2010 data were available from several of the datasets we accessed, major changes in data collection produced marked discontinuity in data output for 2010 versus the prior years. Also, in 2010 there was a jump in the rate of missing data for some important fields, such as source of hospital admission. It will likely take one or two additional years of data collection, and complex statistical adjustments, for analysts to take these differences into account to generate valid longitudinal analyses. For this reason, we restricted the upper end of our study intervals to 2009.

We had hoped to explore the impact of managed care and care coordination on ED admission decisions, but with the exception of the 20 state subsample we examined, the national datasets that are available for public use do not allow researchers to clearly distinguish Medicaid managed care from traditional Medicaid FFS, or private managed care from private FFS. It is possible, if not likely, that large national insurers, such as United Health Group, Cigna, and Aetna can perform such an analysis, but that approach exceeded the resources available for our work.

Our focus groups and interviews were performed with relatively small convenience samples of willing clinicians recruited with the assistance of their respective professional associations and other supportive groups. For this reason, their views may not fully represent the spectrum of provider views on this subject. The dialogue from the three focus groups was recorded but the output was not transcribed. The recordings were used to assure that our interview notes captured all major themes. The individual interviews with PCPs were not recorded. Two team members

53

participated in each session and compared observations to reach agreement, but our analytical approach did not fully comply with the standards articulated in the Qualitative Research Guidelines Project (Cohen & Crabtree, 2006). For this reason, we restricted our qualitative observations to broad consensus themes, with appropriate caveats regarding representativeness.

6. Conclusions

- **EDs are becoming an increasingly important source of hospital admissions.** Since 2003, virtually all of the growth in inpatient admissions was driven by a strong increase in admissions from EDs. This more than offsets a decline in admissions from doctors' offices and other outpatient clinics. By 2009, more than half of all inpatient admissions were entering the hospital through the ED. The strongest growth of inpatient admissions has been among Medicare beneficiaries, six in ten of whom are admitted through the ED. Admissions of privately insured patients have declined, largely because the number of individuals covered by employer-sponsored health insurance declined over the past decade (Institute of Medicine, 2009; White, 2012).

- **Office-based physicians appear to be making growing use of EDs to perform complex workups and expedite non-elective admissions.** The decline of hospital admissions from physicians' offices suggests that some practitioners who previously admitted patients themselves are instead sending these patients to the ED for evaluation and possible admission. Several of the PCPs we interviewed reported that they are increasingly relying on their ED colleagues to facilitate time-urgent workups and non-elective admissions. Our focus group participants offered a variety of justifications for these practices, including illness severity, patient complexity, the patients' need for care after-hours, and the ED physician's access to sophisticated diagnostic equipment that is not available in a doctor's office.

- **ED physicians are serving as the primary decisionmakers for up to half of all hospital admissions.** This estimate is based on the proportion of hospital inpatients being admitted through EDs, and the statements of the PCPs, hospitalists, and emergency physicians whom we interviewed that the physician who evaluates the patient in the ED makes the ultimate decision to admit or discharge.

- **Most patients who visit an ED for a non-emergent health problem do so because they were sent by a health care provider, believed that they had a serious condition, or perceived that they lacked a viable alternative.** CTS data indicate that many primary care practices do not offer after-hours or weekend care, and many surveyed patients perceive that they cannot easily contact their health care provider. Those who do are often advised to seek care in an ED. These findings suggest that efforts to reduce non-urgent visits to EDs should focus on assuring timely access to primary care, rather than blocking access to EDs.

- **Hospital admissions of Medicare patients are growing faster than any other group.** Given their older age and higher prevalence of comorbid conditions, Medicare beneficiaries are more likely to require admission from the ED than Medicaid beneficiaries, privately insured patients, or the uninsured. As the baby boom generation ages and more patients develop chronic conditions, such as diabetes, hypertension, and heart failure, the number of Medicare admissions from EDs will continue to grow.

- **Based on a preliminary analysis of data from 20 states, Medicare beneficiaries covered by a Medicare Advantage plan are less likely to be hospitalized from the ED compared with beneficiaries covered by traditional Medicare FFS.** When the analysis

55

was repeated on a subset of cases with conditions that are considered to be ambulatory care sensitive, a trend towards lower odds of admission among Medicare Advantage patients emerged, but the confidence interval did not exclude 1. Participants in our focus groups and interviews voiced general support for care coordination. Some noted that when a care coordinator is available, they can more confidently discharge a medically fragile patient.

- **Hospital EDs may be playing a constructive role in constraining the growth of potential preventable hospital admissions.** Between 2000 and 2009, ED visits by patients with ACS conditions such as asthma and diabetes increased, but the overall rate of potentially preventable admissions due to these conditions did not. Our analysis strongly suggests, but cannot conclusively prove, that EDs may be helping to constrain the growth of preventable hospital admissions. Further work will be needed to confirm or refute this hypothesis.

Implications for Policy

Hospital EDs serve a number of roles in America's health care system, including serving as a key access point for hospital admissions, a site for conducting complex diagnostic workups, a source of care for patients who cannot get timely access to ambulatory care elsewhere, and a site for non-emergent outpatient care (Smulowitz et al., 2013). In light of these varied roles, hospital administrators, policymakers, payers, and federal research agencies should pay closer attention to ED operations, particularly the role that EDs play in facilitating needed hospital admissions and avoiding those that are preventable.

Likewise, the use of EDs as diagnostic centers warrants further research. There may be considerable benefit to patients and society of facilitating rapid and coordinated assessment of a patient's problem. But it is also possible that assessments conducted in the ED setting are needlessly costly relative to the resulting benefits. In the absence of prospective research, it will be difficult to resolve this question one way or the other. Evidence generated by our study and other published work indicates that efforts to reduce non-emergent and non-urgent use of EDs are most likely to succeed if they focus on providing convenient and affordable options outside the ED, rather than directing ED staff to turn patients away.

All of these efforts can be advanced by achieving more effective integration of EDs into inpatient and outpatient settings. This can be facilitated through more interoperable and interconnected health information technology, greater use of care coordination and case management, and more collaborative approaches to inter-professional practice. More widespread adoption of these and other practice innovations (Smulowitz, 2013) could generate considerable dividends by providing patients with safe and accessible options for non-emergent care; PCPs with ready access to advanced diagnostic resources; ED and hospitalist physicians with the information they need to minimize duplicative testing and avoid needless hospital admissions; and society with better care at lower cost.

References

ACEP. (2013). Washington State is a Model for the Nation, *ACEP Press Release.*

AHRQ. (2012). Quality indicator user guide: Prevention quality indicators (PQI) composite measures, Version 4.4.

AHRQ. (2013). QI SAS®, Version 4.4.

Alhassani, A., Chandra, A., & Chernew, M. E. (2012). The sources of the SGR "hole". *N Engl J Med, 366*(4), 289-291. doi: 10.1056/NEJMp1113059

American College of Emergency Physicians. (2012). Costs of Emergency Care, from http://www.acep.org/content.aspx?id=25902

Amsterdam, E. A., Kirk, J. D., Bluemke, D. A., Diercks, D., Farkouh, M. E., Garvey, J. L., . . . Thompson, P. D. (2010). Testing of low-risk patients presenting to the emergency department with chest pain: a scientific statement from the American Heart Association. *Circulation, 122*(17), 1756-1776. doi: 10.1161/CIR.0b013e3181ec61dfCIR.0b013e3181ec61df [pii]

Apple, F. S., Wu, A. H., Mair, J., Ravkilde, J., Panteghini, M., Tate, J., . . . Jaffe, A. S. (2005). Future biomarkers for detection of ischemia and risk stratification in acute coronary syndrome. *Clin Chem, 51*(5), 810-824. doi: clinchem.2004.046292 [pii] 10.1373/clinchem.2004.046292

Asplin, B. R., Magid, D. J., Rhodes, K. V., Solberg, L. I., Lurie, N., & Camargo, C. A., Jr. (2003). A conceptual model of emergency department crowding. *Ann Emerg Med, 42*(2), 173-180. doi: 10.1067/mem.2003.302S019606440300444X [pii]

Asplin, B. R., Rhodes, K. V., Levy, H., Lurie, N., Crain, A. L., Carlin, B. P., & Kellermann, A. L. (2005). Insurance status and access to urgent ambulatory care follow-up appointments. *JAMA, 294*(10), 1248-1254. doi: 294/10/1248 [pii] 10.1001/jama.294.10.1248

Auerbach, D. I., & Kellermann, A. L. (2011). A decade of health care cost growth has wiped out real income gains for an average US family. *Health Aff (Millwood), 30*(9), 1630-1636. doi: 10.1377/hlthaff.2011.058530/9/1630 [pii]

Baker, L. C. B., L. S. (1994). Excess cost of emergency department visits for nonurgent care. *Health Aff (Millwood), 13*(5), 162-171.

Baugh, C. W., Venkatesh, A. K., & Bohan, J. S. (2011). Emergency department observation units: A clinical and financial benefit for hospitals. *Health Care Manage Rev, 36*(1), 28-37. doi: 10.1097/HMR.0b013e3181f3c03500004010-201101000-00006 [pii]

Begley, C. E., Behan, P., & Seo, M. (2010). Who uses hospital emergency rooms?: Evidence from Houston/Harris County Texas. *J Health Care Poor Underserved, 21*(2), 606-616. doi: 10.1353/hpu.0.0312S1548686910200153 [pii]

Berenson, R. A., & Rich, E. C. (2010). US approaches to physician payment: the deconstruction of primary care. *J Gen Intern Med, 25*(6), 613-618. doi: 10.1007/s11606-010-1295-z

Bernstein, S. L., Aronsky, D., Duseja, R., Epstein, S., Handel, D., Hwang, U., . . . Asplin, B. R. (2009). The effect of emergency department crowding on clinically oriented outcomes. *Acad Emerg Med, 16*(1), 1-10. doi: 10.1111/j.1553-2712.2008.00295.xACEM295 [pii]

Billings, J., Parikh, N., & Mijanovich, T. (2000). Emergency department use in New York City: a substitute for primary care? *Issue Brief (Commonw Fund)*(433), 1-5.

Billings, J., Parikh, N., Mijanovich, T.,. (2000). Emergency room use: The New York Story. *The Commonwealth Fund, 434.*

CDC. (2012). Emergency Room Use Among Adults Aged 18–64: Early Release of Estimates From the National Health Interview Survey, January–June 2011.

Center for Medicare and Medicaid Services. (2012). National Health Care Expenditures Data: National Health Statistics Group.

Readmissions Reduction Program, (2013).

Center for Studying Health System Change. (2013). CTS Physician Surveys and the HSC 2008 Health Tracking Physician Survey.

Cohen, D. J., & Crabtree, B. J. (2006). Qualitative research guidelines project, from http://www.qualres.org/

Community Memorial Hospital. (2012). Intensive CM cuts ED visits, hospitalizations. *Hosp Case Manag, 20*(10), 153-154.

Cutler, D. (2010). How health care reform must bend the cost curve. *Health Aff (Millwood), 29*(6), 1131-1135

Davies, S. M., McDonald, K. M., Schmidt, E., Schultz, E., Geppert, J., & Romano, P. S. (2009). Expanding use of the Prevention Quality Indicators, November 7, 2009: Report of the clinical expert review panel: Agency for Healthcare Research and Quality.

Davis, K. (2011). Health Spending Continues to Moderate, Cost of Reform Overestimated: The Commonwealth fund.

Delia, D., & Cantor, J. C. (2009). Emergency department utilization and capacity. *Synth Proj Res Synth Rep*(17). doi: 4592945929 [pii]

Dennison, C., & Pokras, R. (2000). Design and operation of the National Hospital Discharge Survey: 1998 redesign. *Vital Health Stat, 1*(39).

Devries, A., Li, C. H., & Oza, M. (2013). Strategies to reduce nonurgent emergency department use: experience of a northern virginia employer group. *Med Care, 51*(3), 224-230. doi: 10.1097/MLR.0b013e3182726b83

Elixhauser, A., Steiner, C. A., Whittington, C. et al. (1998). Clinical classifications for health policy research: Hospital inpatient statistics, 1995 *Healthcare Cost and Utilization Project, HCUP 3 Research Note.* Rockville, MD: Agency for Health Care Policy and Research.

Florence, C. S. (2005). Nonurgent care in the emergency department: can we save by shifting the site of care? *Ann Emerg Med, 45*(5), 495-496. doi: S0196064405000028 [pii];10.1016/j.annemergmed.2005.01.001

Flottemesch, T. J., Anderson, L. H., Solberg, L. I., Fontaine, P., & Asche, S. E. (2012). Patient-centered medical home cost reductions limited to complex patients. *Am J Manag Care, 18*(11), 677-686. doi: 80589 [pii]

Fuchs, V. R. (2012). Major Trends in the U.S. Health Economy since 1950. *New England Journal of Medicine, 366*(11), 973-977. doi: doi:10.1056/NEJMp1200478

Gaiser, T. J. (2008). Online focus groups. In N. Fielding, R. M. Lee & G. Blank (Eds.), *The SAGE handbook of online research methods.* London: SAGE.

Ginsburg, P. (2008). High and rising health care costs: Demystifying U.S. health care spending *Research Synthesis Report No. 16.*

Glendenning-Napoli, A., Dowling, B., Pulvino, J., Baillargeon, G., & Raimer, B. G. (2012). Community-based case management for uninsured patients with chronic diseases: effects on acute care utilization and costs. *Prof Case Manag, 17*(6), 267-275. doi: 10.1097/NCM.0b013e3182687f2b01269241-201211000-00005 [pii]

Goodell, S., Delia, D. et Cantor, J.,. (2009). Emergency department utilization and capacity *Policy Brief No.17*: Robert Wood Johnson Foundation.

Graves, E. J. (1995). Detailed diagnoses and procedures, National Hospital Discharge Survey, 1993. In N. C. f. H. Statistics (Ed.), *Vital Health Stat* (Vol. 13(122)).

Healthcare Cost and Utilization Project. (undated). Clinical Classifications Software (CCS) for ICD-9-CM

Hsia, R. Y., Kellermann, A. L., & Shen, Y. C. (2011). Factors associated with closures of emergency departments in the United States. *JAMA, 305*(19), 1978-1985. doi: 10.1001/jama.2011.620305/19/1978 [pii]

Hsia, R. Y., MacIsaac, D., & Baker, L. C. (2008). Decreasing reimbursements for outpatient emergency department visits across payer groups from 1996 to 2004. *Ann Emerg Med, 51*(3), 265-274, 274 e261-265. doi: S0196-0644(07)01436-9 [pii] 10.1016/j.annemergmed.2007.08.009

Institute of Medicine. (2006). IOM report: the future of emergency care in the United States health system. *Acad Emerg Med, 13*(10), 1081-1085. doi: j.aem.2006.07.011 [pii] 10.1197/j.aem.2006.07.011

Institute of Medicine. (2007). Hospital-Based Emergency Care: At the Breaking Point *Consensus Report*.

Institute of Medicine. (2009). Insurance Status and Its Consequences. America's uninsured crisis: consequences for health and health care. *National Academies Press*.

Jaffe, A. S., Babuin, L., & Apple, F. S. (2006). Biomarkers in acute cardiac disease: the present and the future. *J Am Coll Cardiol, 48*(1), 1-11. doi: S0735-1097(06)00920-X [pii] 10.1016/j.jacc.2006.02.056

Jiang, H. J., Russo, C. A., & Barrett, M. L. (2006). Nationwide Frequency and Costs of Potentially Preventable Hospitalizations, 2006: Statistical Brief #72. doi: NBK53971 [bookaccession]

Johnson, P. J., Ghildayal, N., Ward, A. C., Westgard, B. C., Boland, L. L., & Hokanson, J. S. (2012). Disparities in potentially avoidable emergency department (ED) care: ED visits for ambulatory care sensitive conditions. *Med Care, 50*(12), 1020-1028. doi: 10.1097/MLR.0b013e318270bad4

Kaiser Family Foundation. (2012). Employer Health Benefits—2012 Summary of Findings: Menlo Park, Calif.: Kaiser Family Foundation, and Chicago, Ill.: Health Research and Educational Trust.

Kellerman, A. (1994). Access of Medicaid recipients to outpatient care. *N Engl J Med, 330*(20), 1426-1430. doi: 10.1056/NEJM199405193302007

Kellermann, A. L., & Jones, S. S. (2013). What it will take to achieve the as-yet-unfulfilled promises of health information technology. *Health Affairs, 32*(1), 63-68. doi: 10.1377/hlthaff.2012.0693.

Kellermann, A. L., & Martinez, R. (2011). The ER, 50 years on. *N Engl J Med, 364*(24), 2278-2279. doi: 10.1056/NEJMp1101544

Kellermann, A. L. W., R. M. (2012). Emergency departments, Medicaid costs, and access to primary care--understanding the link. *N Engl J Med, 366*(23), 2141-2143. doi: 10.1056/NEJMp1203247

Kharbanda, A. B., Hall, M., Shah, S. S., Freedman, S. B., Mistry, R. D., Macias, C. G., . . . Neuman, M. I. (2013). Variation in Resource Utilization Across a National Sample of Pediatric Emergency Departments. *J Pediatr.* doi: S0022-3476(12)01460-6 [pii] 10.1016/j.jpeds.2012.12.013

Kruzikas, D. T., Jiang, H.J., Remus, D. et al. (2000). Preventable Hospitalizations: A Window Into Primary and Preventive Care: Agency for Healthcare Research and Quality.

Kumar, G. S., & Klein, R. (2012). Effectiveness of Case Management Strategies in Reducing Emergency Department Visits In Frequent User Patient Populations: A Systematic Review. *J Emerg Med.* doi: S0736-4679(12)01120-1 [pii] 10.1016/j.jemermed.2012.08.035

Machlin, S., and Chowdhury,S.,. (2011). Expenses and Characteristics of Physician Visits in Different Ambulatory Care Settings, 2008 (Vol. Statistical Bried #318): Agency for Healthcare Research and Quality.

Martin, A. B., Lassman, D., Washington, B., Catlin, A., & the National Health Expenditure Accounts Team. (2012). Growth in US health spending remained slow 2010; Health share of Gross Domestic Product was unchanged from 2009. *Health Affairs, 31*(1), 208-219.

McKinlay, J. B., & Marceau, L. D. (2012). From cottage industry to a dominant mode of primary care: stages in the diffusion of a health care innovation (retail clinics). *Soc Sci Med, 75*(6), 1134-1141. doi: 10.1016/j.socscimed.2012.04.039S0277-9536(12)00411-X [pii]

McKinsey Global Institute. (2008). Accounting for the cost of U.S. health care: Pre-reform trends and the impact of the recession.

McNeeley, M. F., Gunn, M. L., & Robinson, J. D. (2013). Transfer Patient Imaging: Current Status, Review of the Literature, and the Harborview Experience. *J Am Coll Radiol.* doi: S1546-1440(12)00582-0 [pii] 10.1016/j.jacr.2012.09.031

Mehrotra, A., & Lave, J. R. (2012). Visits to retail clinics grew fourfold from 2007 to 2009, although their share of overall outpatient visits remains low. *Health Aff (Millwood), 31*(9), 2123-2129. doi: 10.1377/hlthaff.2011.1128hlthaff.2011.1128 [pii]

Mehrotra, A., Wang, M. C., Lave, J. R., Adams, J. L., & McGlynn, E. A. (2008). Retail clinics, primary care physicians, and emergency departments: a comparison of patients' visits. *Health Aff (Millwood), 27*(5), 1272-1282. doi: 10.1377/hlthaff.27.5.127227/5/1272 [pii]

Merritt, B., Naamon, E., & Morris, S. A. (2000). The influence of an Urgent Care Center on the frequency of ED visits in an urban hospital setting. *Am J Emerg Med, 18*(2), 123-125.

MetroHealth Medical Center. (2012). Program for uninsured cuts ED visits, admissions. *Hosp Case Manag, 20*(10), 154-155.

Morgan, S. R., Smith, M. A., Pitts, S. R., Shesser, R., Uscher-Pines, L., Ward, M. J., & Pines, J. M. (2012). Measuring value for low-acuity care across settings. *Am J Manag Care, 18*(9), e356-363. doi: 78395 [pii]

O'Mahony, L., O'Mahony, D. S., Simon, T. D., Neff, J., Klein, E. J., & Quan, L. (2013). Medical complexity and pediatric emergency department and inpatient utilization. *Pediatrics, 131*(2), e559-565. doi: 10.1542/peds.2012-1455peds.2012-1455 [pii]

Office of Inspector General. (2012). Coding trends of Medicare Evaluation and Management: Department of Health and Human Services,.

Owens, P. L., Barrett, M. L., Gibson, T. B., Andrews, R. M., Weinick, R. M., & Mutter, R. L. (2010). Emergency department care in the United States: a profile of national data sources. *Ann Emerg Med, 56*(2), 150-165. doi: 10.1016/j.annemergmed.2009.11.022S0196-0644(09)01796-X [pii]

Parmigiani, G., Chen, S., Iversen, E. S., Jr., Friebel, T. M., Finkelstein, D. M., Anton-Culver, H., . . . Euhus, D. M. (2007). Validity of models for predicting BRCA1 and BRCA2 mutations. *Ann Intern Med, 147*(7), 441-450. doi: 147/7/441 [pii]

Pew Center on the States. (2012). State Health Care Spending Project.

Pines, J. M., Mutter, R. L., & Zocchi, M. S. (2013). Variation in Emergency Department Admission Rates Across the United States. *Med Care Res Rev.* doi: 1077558712470565 [pii] 10.1177/1077558712470565

Pitts, S. R. (2012). Higher-complexity ED billing codes--sicker patients, more intensive practice, or improper payments? *N Engl J Med, 367*(26), 2465-2467. doi: 10.1056/NEJMp1211315

Pitts, S. R., Carrier, E. R., Rich, E. C., & Kellermann, A. L. (2010). Where Americans get acute care: increasingly, it's not at their doctor's office. *Health Aff (Millwood), 29*(9), 1620-1629. doi: 10.1377/hlthaff.2009.102629/9/1620 [pii]

Pitts, S. R., Niska, R. W., Xu, J., & Burt, C. W. (2008). National Hospital Ambulatory Medical Care Survey: 2006 emergency department summary. *Natl Health Stat Report*(7), 1-38.

Pitts, S. R., Pines, J. M., Handrigan, M. T., & Kellermann, A. L. (2012). National trends in emergency department occupancy, 2001 to 2008: effect of inpatient admissions versus emergency department practice intensity. *Ann Emerg Med, 60*(6), 679-686 e673. doi: 10.1016/j.annemergmed.2012.05.014S0196-0644(12)00507-0 [pii]

Porter, M. E. (2010). What is value in health care? *N Engl J Med, 363*, 2477-2481.

Porter, M. E., & Teisberg, E. O. (2006). *Redefining health care: Creating value-based competition on results.* Boston: Harvard Business School Press.

Potini, V. C., Weerasuriya, D. N., Lowery-North, D. W., & Kellermann, A. L. (2011). Commercial products that convey personal health information in emergencies. *Disaster Med Public Health Prep, 5*(4), 261-265. doi: 10.1001/dmp.2011.795/4/261 [pii]

Ranseen TA. (1983). Hospital EDs face 'sink-or-swim' time as urgent care center competition rises. Interview by Jean McCann. *Emerg Dep News,, Oct;5(10):1, 6-7,.*

Rasch, E. K., Gulley, S. P., & Chan, L. (2012). Use of Emergency Departments among Working Age Adults with Disabilities: A Problem of Access and Service Needs. *Health Serv Res.* doi: 10.1111/1475-6773.12025

Raven, M. C., Lowe, R. A., Maselli, J., & Hsia, R. Y. (2013). Comparison of presenting complaint vs discharge diagnosis for identifying "nonemergency" emergency department visits. *JAMA, 309*(11), 1145-1153. doi: 10.1001/jama.2013.1948

Reid, R. O., Ashwood, J. S., Friedberg, M. W., Weber, E. S., Setodji, C. M., & Mehrotra, A. (2012). Retail Clinic Visits and Receipt of Primary Care. *J Gen Intern Med.* doi: 10.1007/s11606-012-2243-x

Russo, A., Jiang, H. J., & Barrett, M. (2007). Trends in potentially preventable hospitalizations among adults and children, 1997-2004. In H. C. a. U. Project (Ed.), *Statistical Brief 36*: Agency for Healthcare Research and Quality.

Schuur, J. D., & Venkatesh, A. K. (2012). The growing role of emergency departments in hospital admissions. *N Engl J Med, 367*(5), 391-393. doi: 10.1056/NEJMp1204431

Simonet, D. (2009). Cost reduction strategies for emergency services: insurance role, practice changes and patients accountability. *Health Care Anal, 17*(1), 1-19. doi: 10.1007/s10728-008-0081-0

Smulowitz, P. B., Honigman, L., & Landon, B. E. (2013). A novel approach to identifying targets for cost reduction in the emergency department. *Ann Emerg Med, 61*(3), 293-300. doi: 10.1016/j.annemergmed.2012.05.042

Snell, F. I., Jones, S. L., & Yoder, L. (1987). Factors in choosing an urgent care center versus an emergency department. *J Emerg Nurs, 13*(6), 355-358.

Stranges, E., Kowlessar, N., Elixhauser, A.,. (2011). Components of Growth in Inpatient Hospital Costs, 1997-2009 (Vol. Statistical Bried #123): Agency for Healthcare Research and Quality (AHRQ)

Stubbs, J. W. (2009). Excessive consults stem from lack of time for primary care. *ACP Internist.*

Tang, N., Stein, J., Hsia, R. Y., Maselli, J. H., & Gonzales, R. (2010). Trends and characteristics of US emergency department visits, 1997-2007. *JAMA, 304*(6), 664-670. doi: 10.1001/jama.2010.1112304/6/664 [pii]

Taylor, J. (2006). Don't bring me your tired, your poor: the crowded state of America's emergency departments. *Issue Brief George Wash Univ Natl Health Policy Forum*(811), 1-24.

Taylor, J. (2012). Changes in latitudes, changes in attitudes: FQHCs and community clinics in a reformed health care market. *Issue Brief Natl Health Policy Forum*(848), 1-22.

U.S. Census Bureau. (2012). Statistical Abstract of the United States.

U.S. DHHS. (2009). HCUP Cost-to-Charge Ratio Files (CCR) 2009: Agency for Healthcare Research and Quality.

Uscher-Pines, L., Pines, J., Kellermann, A., Gillen, E., & Mehrotra, A. (2013). Emergency department visits for nonurgent conditions: systematic literature review. *Am J Manag Care, 19*(1), 47-59. doi: 82415 [pii]

Venkatesh, A. K., Geisler, B. P., Gibson Chambers, J. J., Baugh, C. W., Bohan, J. S., & Schuur, J. D. (2011). Use of observation care in US emergency departments, 2001 to 2008. *PLoS One, 6*(9), e24326. doi: 10.1371/journal.pone.0024326PONE-D-11-13459 [pii]

Volpp, K. G., Loewenstein, G., & Asch, D. A. (2012). Choosing wisely: low-value services, utilization, and patient cost sharing. *JAMA, 308*(16), 1635-1636. doi: 10.1001/jama.2012.136161386618 [pii]

Wang, M. C., Ryan, G., McGlynn, E. A., & Mehrotra, A. (2010). Why do patients seek care at retail clinics, and what alternatives did they consider? *Am J Med Qual, 25*(2), 128-134. doi: 10.1177/1062860609353201106286069353201 [pii]

Washington, D. L., Stevens, C. D., Shekelle, P. G., Henneman, P. L., & Brook, R. H. (2002). Next-day care for emergency department users with nonacute conditions. A randomized, controlled trial. *Ann Intern Med, 137*(9), 707-714. doi: 200211050-00005 [pii]

Weber, E. J., Showstack, J. A., Hunt, K. A., Colby, D. C., & Callaham, M. L. (2005). Does lack of a usual source of care or health insurance increase the likelihood of an emergency department visit? Results of a national population-based study. *Ann Emerg Med, 45*(1), 4-12. doi: S0196064404011680 [pii] 10.1016/j.annemergmed.2004.06.023

Weber, E. J., Showstack, J. A., Hunt, K. A., Colby, D. C., Grimes, B., Bacchetti, P., & Callaham, M. L. (2008). Are the uninsured responsible for the increase in emergency department visits in the United States? *Ann Emerg Med, 52*(2), 108-115. doi: 10.1016/j.annemergmed.2008.01.327S0196-0644(08)00365-X [pii]

White, C., Reschovsky, J.,. (2012). Great Recession Accelerated Long-Term Decline of Employer Health Coverage *NIHCR Research Brief No. 8*

Wiler, J. L., Beck, D., Asplin, B. R., Granovsky, M., Moorhead, J., Pilgrim, R., & Schuur, J. D. (2012). Episodes of care: is emergency medicine ready? *Ann Emerg Med, 59*(5), 351-357. doi: 10.1016/j.annemergmed.2011.08.020S0196-0644(11)01544-7 [pii]

Young, G. P., Wagner, M. B., Kellermann, A. L., Ellis, J., & Bouley, D. (1996). Ambulatory visits to hospital emergency departments. Patterns and reasons for use. 24 Hours in the ED Study Group. *JAMA, 276*(6), 460-465.